100 Questions & Answers About Prostate Disease

Kevin R. Loughlin, MD, MBA
Brigham and Women's Hospital
Boston, MA

John Nimmo, BA, MA
Professional Health Strategies, Inc.
Wellesley, MA

JONES AND BARTLETT PUBLISHERS
Sudbury, Massachusetts
BOSTON   TORONTO   LONDON   SINGAPORE

World Headquarters

Jones and Bartlett Publishers	Jones and Bartlett Publishers	Jones and Bartlett Publishers
40 Tall Pine Drive	Canada	International
Sudbury, MA 01776	6339 Ormindale Way	Barb House, Barb Mews
978-443-5000	Mississauga, Ontario	London W6 7PA
info@jbpub.com	L5V 1J2	UK
www.jbpub.com	CANADA	

Jones and Bartlett's books and products are available through most bookstores and online booksellers. To contact Jones and Bartlett Publishers directly, call 800-832-0034, fax 978-443-8000, or visit our website www.jbpub.com.

Substantial discounts on bulk quantities of Jones and Bartlett's publications are available to corporations, professional associations, and other qualified organizations. For details and specific discount information, contact the special sales department at Jones and Bartlett via the above contact information or send an email to specialsales@jbpub.com.

The authors, editor, and publisher have made every effort to provide accurate information. However, they are not responsible for errors, omissions, or for any outcomes related to the use of the contents of this book and take no responsibility for the use of the products described. Treatments and side effects described in this book may not be applicable to all patients; likewise, some patients may require a dose or experience a side effect that is not described herein. The reader should confer with his or her own physician regarding specific treatments and side effects. Drugs and medical devices are discussed that may have limited availability controlled by the Food and Drug Administration (FDA) for use only in a research study or clinical trial. The drug information presented has been derived from reference sources, recently published data, and pharmaceutical research data. Research, clinical practice, and government regulations often change the accepted standard in this field. When consideration is being given to use of any drug in the clinical setting, the health care provider or reader is responsible for determining FDA status of the drug, reading the package insert, reviewing prescribing information for the most up-to-date recommendations on dose, precautions, and contraindications, and determining the appropriate usage for the product. This is especially important in the case of drugs that are new or seldom used.

Library of Congress Cataloging-in-Publication Data
Loughlin, Kevin R.
   100 questions and answers about prostate disease / Kevin R.
Loughlin, John Nimmo.
      p. cm.
   Includes index.
   ISBN-13: 978-0-7637-3142-7 (alk. paper)
   ISBN-10: 0-7637-3142-0 (alk. paper)
   1. Prostate—Diseases—Miscellanea.   I. Nimmo, John. II. Title. III. Title: One hundred questions and answers about prostate disease.
   RC899.L68 2007
   616.6'5—dc22
                                    2006015753

6048

Production Credits
Executive Publisher: Christopher Davis
Production Director: Amy Rose
Production Editor: Carolyn F. Rogers
Associate Editor: Kathy Richardson
Associate Marketing Manager: Laura Kavigian
VP, Manufacturing & Inventory Control: Therese Connell
Composition: Northeast Compositors
Cover Design: Kate Ternullo
Printing and Binding: Malloy, Inc.
Cover Printing: Malloy, Inc.

Printed in the United States of America
10 09 08 07 06   10 9 8 7 6 5 4 3 2 1

Dedication

To my father, the finest man I have known.

KRL

To all my children and grandchildren:
We're learning more every year about what causes and helps to
control diseases, but in spite of the gains, we're still on chapter one.
Keep learning. Help write chapter two!

JN

CONTENTS

Benign prostate hypertrophy, or BPH, is the most common benign disease of older men. Prostate cancer is the most common male cancer and prostatitis is a very common infection. Because of the frequency of these prostatic diseases, almost all men will be faced with some prostatic condition during their lifetime.

Despite the prevalence of prostate disease, controversy abounds over the diagnosis and treatment of prostatic disorders. The purpose of this book, written by a urologist and a patient, is to try to bring order and perspective to what is, at times, the very confusing subject of prostate disease.

PART ONE

The Basics

What does the prostate gland do?

What is the anatomy of the prostate gland?

What diseases can affect the prostate gland?

More . . .

1. Where is the prostate gland?

The **prostate gland** is located at the base of the **bladder**. It surrounds the **urethra**, which is the tube that urine flows through as it passes out the **penis**. The doctor can feel the posterior or back of the prostate through the **rectum**. The anatomy of the prostate is shown in Figure 1.

2. What does the prostate gland do?

The prostate gland accounts for the production of most of the **seminal plasma**, the fluid or ejaculate that carries the **sperm**. Most people do not realize that although the **testicles** produce sperm, the testicles account for

Prostate gland

a male gland that is located at the base of the bladder and surrounds the urethra.

Bladder

the structure in the body that stores urine.

Urethra

the tube that carries urine from the bladder to the outside of the body.

Penis

the male organ used for urination and sexual intercourse.

Rectum

the final, straight portion of the large intestine, ending in the anus.

Seminal plasma

the majority of the ejaculatory fluid that is used to nourish the sperm.

Sperm

the cells in the male ejaculate that fertilize eggs.

Testicles

The reproductive organs of the male, located in the scrotum.

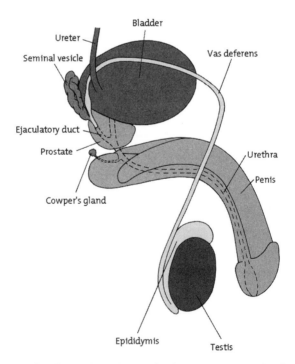

Figure 1   Side view of the male reproductive system. *Source:* Crowley, LV. *An Introduction to Human Disease.* 6th ed. Sudbury, Mass: Jones and Bartlett Publishers; 2004.

only about 1% of the total sperm volume. The prostate gland, the **seminal vesicles**, and the **bulbourethral glands** produce almost all of the ejaculatory volume.

The ejaculatory fluid is believed to help nourish the sperm. The ejaculatory fluid contains a variety of substances, including **prostaglandins**, fructose, citric acid, zinc, and **prostate-specific antigen**.

In addition to these physiologic functions, the size and location of the prostate contributes to the resistance of the flow of urine from the bladder.

3. What is the anatomy of the prostate gland?

As mentioned previously, the prostate gland is situated at the base of the bladder and surrounds the urethra. The prostate tissue is contained within a fibromuscular capsule, much like the skin of an apple that surrounds the pulp. Visually, the prostate is divided into two halves: the right and left lobes. Microscopically, the prostate is subdivided into four areas or zones. The anterior or front of the prostate is called the **anterior fibromuscular stoma**. The area of the prostate that immediately surrounds the urethra is called the **transition zone**. The posterior or back of the prostate is called the **peripheral zone**. The remainder of the prostate that is anterior to or in front of the peripheral zone is referred to as the **central zone**. These prostatic zones are shown in Figure 2.

Seminal vesicles

two structures next to the prostate gland that contribute fluid to the ejaculate.

Bulbourethral glands

two glands that discharge a component of seminal fluid into the urethra; also known as Cowper's glands.

Prostaglandins

chemical messengers made by different organs in the body.

Prostate-specific antigen (PSA)

a chemical made by both benign and malignant prostate tissue. Measurement of PSA serum levels is used as a screening test for prostate cancer.

Anterior fibromuscular stoma

the front of the prostate gland.

Transition zone

the area of the prostate that immediately surrounds the urethra.

Peripheral zone

the posterior or back portion of the prostate.

Central zone

the inner portion of the prostate.

4. What diseases can affect the prostate gland?

Prostatitis

an inflammation or infection of the prostate gland.

Benign prostatic hypertrophy

a benign enlargement of the prostate.

Prostate cancer

the most common male cancer, involving a malignant tumor growth in the prostate gland.

Three diseases can affect the prostate gland: **prostatitis**, **benign prostatic hypertrophy** (BPH), and **prostate cancer**. Prostatitis is an inflammation or infection of the prostate gland. It can affect adult men of any age and is usually treated with antibiotics. The symptoms of prostatitis are variable but often include burning and increased frequency of urination.

BPH is the most common benign disease of males. The onset of benign growth or enlargement of the prostate starts in young adulthood and continues throughout a man's lifetime. As a rough estimate, if you take a man's chronological age in years, that percentage of men at that age will have signs and symptoms of BPH. For example, in a group of 75-year-olds, about three quarters of them will have evidence of BPH.

The symptoms of an enlarged prostate include a decrease in the urinary stream, frequent need for urination, and getting up often at night to urinate.

Cancer of the prostate is the most common male cancer. A male infant born today has about a one in eight chance of developing prostate cancer in his lifetime. This year about 180,000 new cases of prostate cancer will be diagnosed, and about 35,000 men will die from prostate cancer.

Most cases of prostate cancer do not present with symptoms but are diagnosed by a rectal exam, a blood test known as prostate-specific antigen (PSA), or a combination of the two.

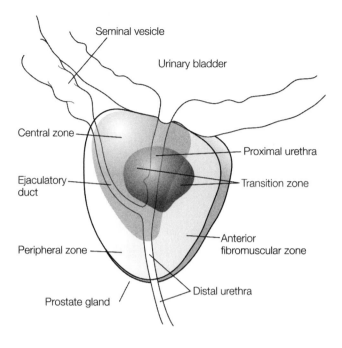

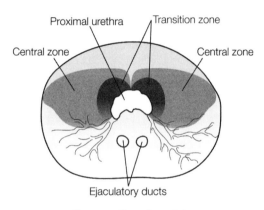

Cross section of prostate

Figure 2   Zones of the prostate. *Source:* **Kirby R, McConnell JD, Fitzpatrick JM, Roehrborn CG, Boyle P, eds.** *Textbook of Benign Prostatic Hyperplasia.* **Oxford, England: Isis Medical Media; 1996.**

PART TWO

Prostate- Specific Antigen (PSA)

What is PSA?

What is the normal range of PSA?

What factors can influence PSA levels?

More . . .

5. What is PSA?

Serine protease

a class of peptidases found in the blood.

PSA is a **serine protease** that was originally identified and isolated in the seminal plasma. The physiologic role of PSA is the liquefaction of semen. PSA is made by both benign and cancerous (malignant) prostate tissue, although malignant prostate tissue makes about 20 times more PSA per gram than benign tissue. Therefore, an elevation of serum PSA can be seen with either benign or malignant growth of the prostate. For all intents and purposes, PSA is made only by prostate tissue and not by any other cells in the body. PSA has therefore gained widespread use as a tumor marker to aid in the diagnosis and management of prostate cancer.

JN: Is PSA the only marker in the blood that signals the possibility of prostate cancer?

KL: Yes.

6. What is the normal range of PSA?

PSA is measured as a blood test. Many, but not all, physicians feel that measuring PSA on a regular basis picks up prostate cancer earlier and saves lives; however, considerable debate still exists within the medical community about whether PSA screening is useful. Those who endorse PSA screening recommend that men over the age of 50 years get a PSA test and a rectal exam annually. Screening advocates recommend that the annual PSA test commence at the age of 40 years in high-risk groups such as men with a family history of prostate cancer or African American men.

The normal range of PSA is considered to be between 0 and 4 ng/ml.

7. What are age-adjusted PSA ranges?

The concept of age-adjusted PSA ranges is based on two observations: first that both benign and malignant growth of the prostate result in elaboration of PSA and second that as men get older their prostate gets larger. Therefore, in general, as men age, their overall PSA levels increase. Age-adjusted PSA ranges result in lower normal ranges for younger men and higher normal ranges for older men. This results in a lower threshold to initiate an evaluation in younger men and a higher threshold for evaluation in older men. This should result in two benefits. First, prostate cancer would be diagnosed more readily in younger men, and second, it would prompt fewer biopsies in older men. The commonly accepted age-adjusted PSA ranges appear in Table 1. There are no age-adjusted PSA ranges for men in their 80s, as most physicians do not feel that men in that age group benefit by being screened for prostate cancer.

Table 1 Age-adjusted PSA ranges

Age (yrs)	PSA Normal Range (ng/ml)
40–49	0.0–2.5
50–59	0.0–3.5
60–69	0.0–4.5
70–79	0.0–6.5

Prostate-Specific Antigen (PSA)

JN: Researchers at the University of Michigan Medical School have discovered a gene that holds a clue as to whether a prostate cancer will develop into its most fast-acting, aggressive form. In the metastatic cells that the researchers examined, a gene designated as EZH2 was found to be most active. Patients with higher levels of EZH2 were more likely to get the lethal form of prostate cancer, causing the scientists to suggest that EZH2 may be a more accurate measurement of a patient's blood than PSA.

KL: There is active research to identify genetic markers for prostate cancer, but none of these markers is currently used clinically.

8. What is PSA density?

PSA density

a measurement calculated by dividing the serum PSA by the prostate volume.

Like age-adjusted PSA values, the concept of **PSA density** is based on the knowledge that although both benign and malignant prostate tissue make PSA, malignant prostate tissue makes more per gram. Therefore, the greater density of PSA per total volume of a prostate, the greater likelihood that prostate will contain some cancer. Several studies have evaluated this concept. The serum PSA was measured in a group of men and their prostate volume in grams was estimated by a transrectal ultrasound by dividing the serum PSA by the prostate volume. The men most likely to have cancer had PSA density volumes greater than 0.15. One practical drawback from using PSA density clinically is that it requires a patient to go through a **transrectal ultrasound**, which is somewhat uncomfortable.

Transrectal ultrasound

a prodecure in which a probe is placed in the rectum to visualize the prostate.

9. What is PSA velocity?

PSA velocity refers to the change in PSA levels over time. It has been published that a change of PSA of greater than 0.75 ng/ml over an interval of 1 year is worrisome for prostate cancer and merits a prostate biopsy. This change of a 0.75 ng/ml is an absolute value and applies regardless of the baseline PSA value. Therefore, a change of PSA from 4.0 to 4.8 ng/ml carries the same import as a change of PSA from 8.0 to 8.8 ng/ml. It should be recognized that the concept of PSA velocity was an outgrowth of a retrospective study that measured PSA levels in the stored blood samples of men who had been followed over a period of years. The PSA values of the stored samples were run several times, and averages were calculated; therefore, it is not totally valid to use a single PSA value taken in year 2 and compare its change with a single PSA value from year 1, as is usually done in clinical practice. In addition, there are differences in the PSA assays that are used in different hospitals and laboratories that make comparison of PSA values obtained at different institutions unwieldy in calculating PSA velocity.

PSA velocity
the change in the PSA level over time.

10. What is free PSA?

For reasons that are not totally understood, PSA that is made by prostate cancer cells is preferentially bound to a serum protein known as **alpha-1-antichymotrypsin**, whereas PSA elaborated by benign prostate cells is free or unbound. Most laboratories now provide the fraction of free PSA as a percentage of the total PSA. Again, assays may vary from laboratory to laboratory, but generally, a free fraction of 25 percent or more is considered consistent with benign disease.

Alpha-1-antichymotrypsin
substance in the blood that can bind PSA.

JN: When a patient has a PSA test of his blood, should he always ask his doctor to include a test of free PSA and complex PSA?

KL: No, this should be left up to the judgment of the urologist. Calculations of free PSA are most useful in men who have had an elevated PSA in the past with negative biopsies. If the total PSA remains elevated and the free PSA fraction is depressed, the urologist is more likely to recommend a repeat biopsy.

11. What is complexed PSA?

Complexed PSA

PSA that is bound to alpha-1-antichy-motrypsin.

Complexed PSA is an assay that measures the PSA that is bound to alpha-1-antichymotrypsin. In a sense, it is the converse of free PSA. Some reports have advocated the use of complexed PSA to help differentiate cancer of the prostate from BPH; however, its superiority to the standard total and free PSA calculations has not been conclusively proven. In addition, not all laboratories offer complexed PSA measurements.

12. What is HK2?

Human glandular kallikrein

a substance made by the prostate gland that is not used as a tumor marker.

Human glandular kallikrein (HK2) was first isolated from seminal plasma in the ejaculate. HK2 is similar to but distinct from PSA. Some experimental studies have demonstrated that HK2 measurements may be helpful in differentiating malignant from benign prostate disease; however, the role of HK2 is not fully understood, and its measurement is only available through certain research facilities. It is not currently used clinically.

13. What is acid phosphatase?

Acid phosphatase

tumor marker for prostate cancer that is no longer used.

Acid phosphatase is an enzyme found in the blood that is made primarily by the prostate gland. Before the PSA era, it was the only prostate cancer marker available, and like PSA, acid phosphatase is made by both benign and malignant prostate tissue; however, acid phosphatase levels can vary markedly and are not as reliable a marker as PSA. Acid phosphatase is no longer used today in the diagnosis and management of prostate cancer.

14. What factors can influence PSA levels?

Several factors can affect PSA levels and cause false elevations of a PSA reading. An infection of the prostate, known as **prostatitis**, can cause a transient elevation of serum PSA. The symptoms of prostatitis can include burning with urination, frequency of urination, pain with ejaculation, or blood in the semen known as **hematospermia**. When a patient is suspected of having prostatitis, a PSA level should not be drawn, as it can be falsely elevated.

A prostate biopsy will also cause a temporary increase in the PSA level. Therefore, if for some reason a repeat PSA level is desired after a patient has had a prostate biopsy, a repeat PSA should not be drawn for at least 6 weeks after the biopsy. A rectal exam or an ejaculation may cause a mild rise of PSA, but not enough to cause a normal value to increase into the abnormal range; therefore, a patient can have a PSA level drawn after his physician has examined him or after he has ejaculated. A **cystoscopy**, or looking into the bladder with a special instrument inserted through the penis, usually does not cause a significant change in the PSA level, but most urologists prefer to obtain the PSA value prior to the cystoscopy.

Prostatitis

an inflammation or infection of the prostate gland

Hematospermia

the presence of blood in ejaculate (semen).

Cystoscopy

a procedure to look into the bladder and urethra with a special tube.

Prostate-Specific Antigen (PSA)

13

PART THREE

Benign Prostatic Hypertrophy (BPH)

What are the symptoms of BPH?

How is BPH diagnosed?

What is the relationship between BPH and PSA?

More ...

15. What causes BPH?

The short answer is that no one knows for sure. The growth of the prostate gland is a complex process that starts at puberty and continues throughout adult life. As a man ages, his prostate grows, although the rate of growth and size of the prostate varies from individual to individual. It is certain that prostate growth, whether it is benign or malignant, requires **testosterone**. Centuries ago, it was observed that the castrati, the Italian opera singers who were castrated at puberty to preserve their tenor voices, never developed enlargement of their prostates.

As more has been understood about the benign growth of the prostate, it has been discovered that testosterone is converted to a substance called **dihydrotestosterone** (DHT), which directly acts on the prostate and mediates benign enlargement. Other growth factors may be involved in addition to DHT, and research is continuing in this area.

Testosterone

the principal male sex hormone.

Dihydrotestosterone

a metabolite of testosterone.

16. How common is BPH?

BPH is the most common disease of mankind. It has been said that if a man lives long enough, he will develop BPH; however, autopsy studies have shown that some men, even in their 30s, have anatomic evidence for significant prostate enlargement. The degree of prostatic enlargement is variable; however, the following numbers are useful guidelines. At the age of 30 years, an average prostate size is 20 grams; by age 70 years, the average prostate size is 35 grams.

As an estimate, if you take a man's chronologic age in years, roughly that percentage of men at that age will have signs of BPH; however, importantly, there is not a linear correlation between prostate size and prostate symptoms. Some men with relatively small glands will have significant symptoms, whereas some men with large glands will have minimal symptoms.

17. What are the symptoms of BPH?

An enlarged prostate can cause a variety of symptoms. Some are referred to as obstructive symptoms and include weak stream, hesitancy of voiding, intermittent stream, a sensation of incomplete bladder emptying, and terminal dribbling. Irritative symptoms include frequent urination, **nocturia** (getting up at night to urinate), and the urge to urinate.

Other conditions that may be a sign of prostatic enlargement are urinary retention or the inability to void, urinary tract infection, **urinary incontinence**, and **hematuria** or blood in the urine.

It is important to acknowledge that bladder dysfunction can either mimic or contribute to some of these symptoms, and the physician must consider these when a diagnosis of prostatic enlargement is made.

JN: There are ads that promote a pill that controls an "overactive bladder." Could a pill that controls overactive bladders be helpful to men with BPH in reducing frequency?

KL: Yes, that is why it is important for the urologist to differentiate between BPH and an overactive bladder.

Nocturia

getting up at night to urinate.

Urinary incontinence

leakage of urine from the bladder through the urethra.

Hematuria

the presence of blood in urine.

18. How is BPH diagnosed?

Both a physical exam and history are used to diagnose BPH. When necessary, the **urologist** may use other diagnostic tests to obtain additional information to help make the diagnosis.

If a patient gives a history that includes one or more of the symptoms mentioned in Question 17, the physician will be alerted to consider BPH as part of his differential diagnosis. Also, when the physician performs a **digital rectal exam** (palpates or feels the prostate with a finger in the rectum), he or she can feel whether the prostate is enlarged.

Finally, if the physician needs additional information before making a diagnosis of BPH, he or she can do additional tests, which include a **uroflow**, a **bladder ultrasound**, a **cystoscopy**, and a **urodynamics test**.

19. What is a uroflow measurement?

A uroflow measurement is a totally noninvasive test. The patient, with a full bladder, voids into a special urinal that has a flowmeter, which measures both the urine flow in milliliters per second as well as the total volume voided. This is plotted onto a piece of paper, and there are nomograms available that allow the doctor to compare the patient's urine flow with accepted standards. The uroflow is typically done in the physician's office at the time of the patient's visit.

20. What is a bladder ultrasound?

A bladder ultrasound is performed by placing an ultrasound probe, which is like a plastic microphone, on the patient's lower abdomen over the bladder. This is done

Urologist

a person trained to treat the genitourinary system.

Digital rectal exam

part of the physical exam where the urologist palpates the prostate by inserting a finger into the rectum.

Uroflow

a measurement of the force and volume of the urine stream.

Bladder ultrasound

a test done through the skin to measure how much urine is left in the bladder after voiding.

Cystoscope

the instrument that is used to look into the bladder during a cystoscopy.

Urodynamics test

a test that assesses how well the bladder functions.

after the patient has been asked to void, and the probe calculates how much urine is left in the bladder. This procedure is totally painless, and a medical assistant, a nurse, or a physician performs this in a physician's office.

21. What is a cystoscopy?

Cystoscopy means literally to look into the bladder. A cystoscope is either a rigid or flexible instrument that has a lens at one end and is connected to a light source. The instrument permits the urologist to look up through the penis and through the prostate and into the bladder. A cystoscopy can be done with either a rigid or flexible cystoscope. If a rigid cystoscope is used, the patient is placed on his back with his feet in stirrups (Figure 3). If a flexible cystoscope is used, the patient is positioned flat on his back with his feet out straight or the supine position. A cystoscopy can be

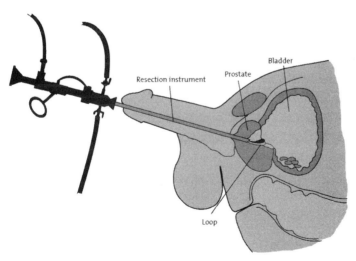

Figure 3 Position for cystoscopy. *Source:* Crowley, LV. *An Introduction to Human Disease.* 6th ed. Sudbury, Mass: Jones and Bartlett Publishers; 2004.

performed with either the patient under general spinal or local anesthesia and can be done in either the physician's office or the operating room in the hospital.

22. What is a urodynamics test?

A urodynamics test is a way to assess the function of the bladder. It can also measure the degree of blockage or obstruction that the prostate is causing. In a sense, a urodynamics test does for the bladder what an ECG or electrocardiogram does for the heart. It tells you how well the bladder muscle is working.

A urodynamics test is always done with the patient awake because it is interactive. The patient has to tell the doctor or nurse performing the test what he is feeling (e.g., does his bladder feel full, and does he feel the urge to void?).

Catheter

a soft plastic or rubber tube that is inserted in the urethra, through the prostate, and into the bladder in order to drain urine.

The urodynamics test is pretty straightforward. The patient lies on his back, and his genitals are washed with a sterile solution; then sterile drapes are placed around the genitals. A rubber **catheter** is placed through the penis into the bladder, and the catheter is connected to a machine that records pressure measurements. Fluid is run through the catheter into the bladder to mimic the bladder being filled with urine. During the urodynamics test, x-rays of the bladder can also be taken. A typical urodynamics test usually takes 45 minutes to 1 hour to perform.

JN: Apart from frequency, what sort of symptoms would a patient usually have to make the doctor call for an urodynamics test?

KL: Nocturia, decreased force of stream, urgency, or incontinence.

23. What is the relationship between BPH and PSA?

As mentioned previously, benign prostate tissue makes PSA, although not as much per gram as malignant prostate tissue. Therefore, as the prostate grows, the PSA level increases. An elevated PSA can therefore signify either an underlying prostate malignancy or benign growth of the prostate. In men with a mild elevation of their PSA (4 to 10 ng/dl), approximately 25% of the biopsies will be positive for cancer, but 75% will not.

24. What other disorders can mimic BPH?

Other underlying disorders can mimic the symptoms of BPH. A **neurogenic bladder**, or bladder with impairment of its nerve supply, can cause a patient to void either frequently or infrequently depending on the nature of the neurologic problem. At times, a neurogenic bladder can cause the patient to be unable to urinate or go into urinary retention.

Diabetes mellitus can cause frequent urination, as many patients with diabetes make a greater volume of urine per 24 hours. With long-standing diabetes, bladder damage can occur that results in a decreased ability of the bladder to contract and therefore causes less frequent urination.

A urinary tract infection can cause urinary frequency and burning with urination. A urethral stricture or scar

Neurogenic bladder

a bladder that has an abnormality in its nerve supply.

Diabetes mellitus

a disorder in which blood sugar (glucose) levels are abnormally high because the body does not produce enough insulin.

tissue in the urethra from old infections or trauma can cause a decrease in the urinary stream.

25. What damage can BPH cause?

One way to think of BPH is that it is causing increased resistance to the flow of urine out of the bladder. This can result in a transmission of back pressure to the bladder and ultimately to the kidneys.

Bladder stones

hard buildups of mineral that form in the urinary bladder.

Men with long-standing prostatic obstruction and incomplete bladder emptying can form **bladder stones**, which can result in bleeding and infection. With significant and chronic prostatic obstruction, the bladder can be damaged and not contract well, much like if you chronically overinflated the inner tube of a tire.

Azotemia

increased serum creatinine which is a sign of kidney dysfunction.

Finally, some men with chronic prostatic obstruction can develop kidney damage known as **azotemia** because of the long-standing back pressure that is transmitted to the kidneys.

JN: Are there symptoms that a patient with BPH should be aware of that would signal the likelihood of his condition worsening to the point where he would experience acute urinary retention?

KL: Not necessarily, unfortunately, urinary retention can occur without warning.

JN: If BPH can cause increased resistance to the flow of urine from the bladder and transmission of back pressure to the bladder and ultimately to the kidneys, is there any way a patient would recognize symptoms that would signal him to know that his enlarged prostate was now starting to cause bladder and possible kidney problems? If undetected, could the kidney problems develop into renal failure?

KL: Symptoms cannot predict kidney problems and which men may be at risk for renal failure. A blood test called serum creatinine is the best way to assess kidney function.

26. Does nutrition have any impact on BPH?

For many years, it has been known that the prostate has the highest concentration of zinc of any organ in the body. Therefore, the conventional wisdom has said that zinc supplements are good for the prostate; however, very little objective evidence exists that zinc prevents either enlargement of the prostate or cancer of the prostate. If zinc supplements are beneficial to the prostate, no one knows the optimal dose. Most multivitamin preparations available in any drugstore, however, contain variable amounts of zinc.

There has also been increasing interest in herbal therapy to treat benign enlargement of the prostate. Saw palmetto is the most popular herb used to treat BPH, and some studies have shown a benefit from saw palmetto. Like zinc, however, no one knows what the optimal dose of saw palmetto is. We go into further detail regarding herbal therapy in Question 41.

In general, nutrition and its impact on BPH have been understudied, and much more work needs to be done regarding the relationship between diet and prostate disease.

PART FOUR

Medical Treatment of Benign Prostatic Hypertrophy

When does BPH need to be treated?

How are alpha blockers used to treat BPH symptoms?

What are the results of BPH treatment using 5 alpha reductase inhibitor drugs?

More ...

27. When does BPH need to be treated?

The need to initiate treatment for BPH is divided into absolute and relative indications. Absolute indications refer to objective medical reasons to intervene. These include impaired renal function because of prostatic obstruction, **hydronephrosis** or dilation of the ureters and kidneys, recurrent urinary tract infections, and bladder stones.

Hydronephrosis
dilation of the kidneys, usually due to obstruction.

These absolute and relative indications for the treatment of BPH appear in Table 2.

Impaired renal function, hydronephrosis or dilation of the drainage system of the kidney, recurrent urinary tract infections, bladder stones, and urinary retention are considered absolute indications for intervention. These conditions are considered absolute because if left untreated they can cause harm to the patient.

The relative indications refer to symptoms that may or may not be bothersome to an individual patient. These include urinary frequency, nocturia (getting up at night to urinate), and decreased urinary stream. The reason that these are referred to as relative indications is that not all symptoms bother patients

Table 2   Indications for BPH treatment

Absolute	Relative
Impaired renal function	Nocturia
Hydronephrosis	Urinary frequency
Recurrent UTIs	Urinary urgency
Bladder stones	Decreased force of stream
Urinary retention	

equally. For instance, getting up three times per night may bother one man a great deal and another not at all. Therefore, whether to treat these relative symptoms depends in large measure by how much they bother the individual patients.

28. What are alpha receptors, and how do they influence BPH symptoms?

Alpha receptors are the nerve fibers that mediate bladder and prostate function and tone. Alpha receptors, however, are found throughout the body, and they control a variety of physiologic functions, not just voiding. Alpha receptors respond to **norepinephrine**, which is a **neurotransmitter**. Alpha receptors are found in what is known as the sympathetic nervous system. When norepinephrine reaches the alpha receptors, it causes a change in the tone of smooth muscle fibers.

There are three distinct types of alpha receptors: alpha 1a, alpha 1b, and alpha 1d. They have different distributions throughout the body. Alpha 1a receptors are found in very high concentrations within the prostatic smooth muscle and therefore are very important in regulating prostatic tone. Alpha 1b receptors play a relatively minor role in the urinary tract and are found primarily in the central nervous system, spleen, and lungs. Alpha 1d receptors are the predominant alpha receptors found in the smooth muscle of the bladder. Alpha 1a and alpha 1b receptors are also found in vascular smooth muscle throughout the body.

When alpha receptors in the prostatic smooth muscle are stimulated by norepinephrine, the result is increased tone of the prostatic smooth muscle. A way

Alpha receptors
the nerve fibers that mediate bladder and prostate function and tone.

Norepinephrine
a neurotransmitter that regulates the sympathetic nervous system.

Neurotransmitter
chemicals that influence the function of nerves.

to think of this is that the prostate squeezes around the urethra and tightens its grip, resulting in increased urethral resistance to urine flow from the bladder. This increased prostatic tone, therefore, can result in the symptoms of prostatic obstruction.

29. How are alpha blockers used to treat BPH symptoms?

Because norepinephrine is the signal that acts on the alpha receptors to cause smooth muscle to contract, if you block part of that signal, you should decrease the muscle contraction. This is the underlying rationale for the use of a class of drugs known as **alpha blockers** to treat obstructive urinary symptoms.

Alpha blockers

a class of drug used to treat prostate symptoms.

Many alpha blockers are available as oral agents that are readily absorbed by the body and then competitively bind the alpha receptors, which prevent some of the uptake of norepinephrine.

30. What alpha-blocker drugs are available for BPH symptoms?

Over the past decade, an increasing number of alpha blockers have become available on the U.S. market. They are generally divided into specific and nonspecific alpha blockers, depending on which receptors they block, as mentioned in Question 28. Specific alpha blockers act primarily on the prostate with fewer systemic effects. Nonspecific alpha blockers act both systemically and on the prostate. A summary of the currently available alpha blockers and their characteristics appears in Table 3.

Table 3   Currently available alpha blockers

Drug: Generic (Brand Name)	Receptors	Dose (mg)
Phenoxybenzamine (Dibenzyline)	∝1a ∝ 1b ld ∝2a ∝2b ∝2c ∝2d	20–40, 2–3 times/day
Alfuzosin (Uroxatral)	∝ la ∝ 1b 1d	10, once per day
Doxazosin (Cardura)	∝ la ∝ 1b ∝ 1d	4–8, once per day
Prazosin (Minipress)	∝ la ∝ 1b ∝ 1d	1, twice per day
Terazosin (Hytrin)	∝ la ∝1b ∝ 1d	2–10, once per day
Tamsulosin (Flomax)	∝ la ∝ 1d	0.4–0.8, once per day

The patient and his doctor should choose which alpha blocker to use. This will depend on whether the patient has other illnesses, such as hypertension, that can be treated with alpha blockers as well. In addition, the use of some alpha blockers is relatively contraindicated when the patient is taking certain **impotence** medications.

JN: What other known medications might affect any of the medications a patient takes to treat BPH or prostate cancer?

KL: There are potential interactions between the alpha blockers and the oral impotence drugs such as Viagra, Levitra, and Cialis. A patient who is on an alpha blocker should check with his urologists before starting one of the impotence drugs.

JN: Can alpha blockers or any drug create an imbalance with other substances that the body produces such as proteins, amino acids, and enzymes that would alter the normal production of these substances, such as the way

Impotence

the inability to achieve an erection or to maintain an erection until ejaculation.

aspirin affects the formation of platelets or the way Prilosec cuts down on stomach acids?

KL: No, alpa blockers do not create chemical imbalances in the body.

31. What are the side effects of alpha-blocker drugs?

The side effects of alpha-blocker drugs are due primarily to blockade of alpha receptor sites outside of the urinary tract. Commonly reported side effects of alpha-blocker drugs include dizziness, headache, asthenia (weakness), **postural hypotension** (decreased blood pressure with change of body position), **rhinitis** (inflammation of nasal mucous membranes), and ejaculatory dysfunction. These side effects occur in about 5% to 9% of patients taking the drugs and can be reversed by stopping the drugs.

Postural hypotension

a drop in blood pressure upon standing.

Rhinitis

an inflammation of the nasal passages.

32. What are the results of BPH treatment using alpha-blocker drugs?

All six of the alpha blockers commonly used today in the United States have been demonstrated to be beneficial in the treatment of prostatic obstruction; however, both Phenoxybenzamine (Dibenzyline) and Prazosin (Minipress) are not commonly used anymore because to be effective they have to be taken more than once per day.

Terazosin (Hytrin) was studied in a randomized, placebo-controlled fashion and was found to be very effective in treating the symptoms of BPH. Two hundred eighty-five patients were entered into a study where placebo, or different doses of terazosin were given. Response rates were evaluated using subjective measures (symptoms were improved) and objective measures (urinary flow rate).

The percentages of patients exhibiting a greater than 30% improvement in symptom scores and flow rates appear in Figure 4 (adapted from *Textbook of Benign Prostatic Hyperplasia*, Kirby et al.).

Doxazosin (Cardura) has also been proven to be efficacious in the treatment of BPH. Five double-blind, placebo-controlled clinical studies of doxazosin have been published in the literature. These studies demonstrated that doxazosin improved objective measurements such as flow rates, as well as subjective measurements such as symptom scores.

Tamsulosin (Flomax) is a more selective alpha blocker than either terazosin or doxazosin. It therefore has a

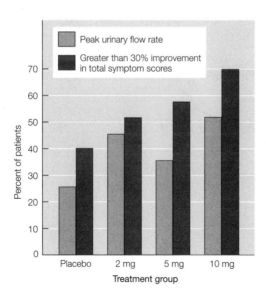

Figure 4   Symptom scores and flow rates. *Source:* Kirby R, McConnell JD, Fitzpatrick JM, Roehrborn CG, Boyle P, eds. *Textbook of Benign Prostatic Hyperplasia*. Oxford, England: Isis Medical Media; 1996.

lower systemic side-effect profile than terazosin or doxazosin. Like other alpha blockers, tamsulosin has a low incidence of dizziness (5.7%), hypotension (0.4%), or fainting (0.2%).

Alpha blocker drugs have been proven effective in treating the symptoms that are often associated with an enlarged prostate. Whenever you gauge the effectiveness of any therapy for the treatment of prostate symptoms, it is important to have a control group, as there is often a significant placebo effect observed in the treatment of prostatism. It is important to recognize that symptom score improvement is a subjective measure based on the patient's perception as to whether his symptoms have improved after taking a drug. The peak flow rate is an objective measure based on the force of the patient's urinary stream measured by a machine. Alpha blockers have been shown to be efficacious in the treatment of obstructive prostate disease by both objective and subjective measures. To date, no study has yet shown that alpha blockers reduce the risk of going into urinary retention.

33. What is DHT?

DHT is a metabolite of testosterone that mediates secondary sexual characteristics, including prostate growth. The major male hormone, testosterone, is converted into DHT by an enzyme known as 5 alpha reductase. 5 alpha reductase was discovered independently in 1974 by Julianne Imperato-McGinley and Patrick Walsh. Julianne Imperato-McGinley was actually studying children in Santo Domingo with ambiguous genitalia and noted that when the male children grew up they never developed enlarged prostates. It was her work and that by

Patrick Walsh that established that DHT was the active agent that mediated prostate growth.

Testosterone governs libido or sex drive and to some degree erectile function. It controls the growth of the prostate indirectly as it is converted by 5 alpha reductase into DHT. A schema that depicts the action of 5 alpha reductase appears in Figure 5.

34. What types of 5 alpha reductase inhibitors are available?

The enzymes 5 alpha reductase are present in two iso-forms: type 1 and type 2. Type 1 is found predominantly in extra prostatic tissues such as the skin and liver, although it is also found in the prostate. Type 2 is found predominantly in the prostate. Two drugs have been developed that inhibit 5 alpha reductase. The first is finasteride or Proscar, which is a type 2 or selective 5 alpha reductase inhibitor. The second is dutasteride or Avodart, which is a type 1 and type 2 or nonselective 5 alpha reductase inhibitor. Finasteride has been shown to reduce serum DHT levels by 70%, whereas dutasteride has been shown to reduce serum DHT by 90%. It is not yet known whether that difference in DHT suppression translates into greater efficacy for the patient.

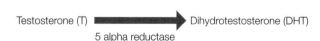

Figure 5 **Action of 5 alpha reductase**

JN: Because Proscar can cut a patient's PSA levels by 50%, wouldn't this also help to cut the patient's risk of prostate cancer by 50%?

KL: Currently, it is not known with certainty whether either finasteride or dutasteride can prevent the development of prostate cancer. Studies are ongoing to answer this question.

35. What are the side effects of 5 alpha reductase inhibitors?

Alpha receptors are found in tissues throughout the body; therefore, alpha blockers can cause side effects or symptoms not related to voiding. A variety of side effects have been reported with the use of alpha blockers for voiding dysfunction. These include dizziness, headache, postural hypotension, drowsiness, tachycardia (fast heart rate), skin rashes, dry mouth, diarrhea, nausea, vomiting, asthenia (weakness), chest pain, and erectile dysfunction. These side effects are rare, but the patient should discuss possible side effects fully with his doctor before starting an alpha blocker for voiding problems. In addition, alpha blockers can interact with some other drugs, particularly those used to treat high blood pressure, and these potential drug interactions should also be discussed with the treating physician.

JN: If a 5 alpha reductase inhibitor such as Proscar (finasteride) does block the conversion of testosterone into DHT and a patient taking Proscar finds his prostate continuing to grow, what other known substances might have a role in the growth of the prostate?

KL: DHT appears to be the driving force causing prostatic growth; however, a variety of other growth factors may play a minor role as well.

36. What are the results of BPH treatment using 5 alpha reductase inhibitor drugs?

As mentioned previously, finasteride (Proscar) and dutasteride (Avodart) are the two 5 alpha reductase inhibitors that are currently available in the United States. Both of these drugs require 3 to 6 months to see clinical beneficial effects. The Finasteride Study Group showed improvement in peak flow rates and symptom scores as well as a decrease in prostate volume. At 1 year, patients on 5 milligrams of finasteride had a 22% improvement in peak flow rates and a 21% decrease in symptom scores. In addition, they exhibited a 19% decrease in their prostate volume.

A recent report looking at cohort of patients treated with dutasteride showed similar improvement in urinary flow rates, a decrease in symptom scores, and a reduction in prostate volume.

37. What effects do 5 alpha reductase inhibitor drugs have on PSA levels?

PSA is a valuable blood test that screens for prostate cancer, as discussed in Questions 5 to 11. However, 5 alpha reductase inhibitor drugs do affect PSA levels.

As mentioned in Question 33, 5 alpha reductase inhibitor drugs block the conversion of testosterone to DHT, which results in shrinkage of the prostate or a decrease in prostate volume. Because prostate cells make PSA, it is reasonable to assume that as the prostate gets smaller, the PSA level will decline. This is in fact what happens; however, it takes 3 to 6 months for a significant volume decrease to occur, and thus, the PSA decline is gradual. Nonetheless, by about 6 months after starting a 5 alpha reductase inhibitor, the total PSA level is about half of the baseline value. The free fraction of PSA is not changed by treatment with 5 alpha reductase inhibitors.

This influence of 5 alpha reductase inhibitors on PSA does not diminish the usefulness of PSA in managing patients with prostate disease. For example, if a 65-year-old man has been on a 5 alpha reductase inhibitor for 6 months, a PSA is drawn, and the value returns as 3.2 ng/ml with 22% free fraction; a simple doubling of the total value to 6.4 ng/ml is made, and the free fraction remains unchanged at 22%. The clinician and patient can then react to the 6.4, 22% value, as would be their custom with any other patient in that age range.

38. Can alpha blocker drugs and 5 alpha reductase drugs be used together?

The short answer to this question is yes. For several years, many urologists used these drugs together with the rationale that because their mechanisms of action were different, their benefits might be additive; however, there was no objective proof that this really was so. A recent study, known as the MTOPS (The Medical Therapy of Prostate Symptoms) study, was published in the *New England Journal of Medicine* (2003;349). It looked at whether a combination of both kinds of drugs was better than either drug alone.

This study was a double-blind trial that involved over 3,000 men who were followed for an average of 4.5 years. The men were divided into four groups: placebo (control group), doxazosin (an alpha blocker) alone, finasteride alone, and doxazosin and finasteride together. These four groups of patients were then followed for signs of progression of BPH. Progression was defined as an increase of urinary symptoms, as measured by the American Urological Association symptom score, acute urinary retention, urinary incontinence, renal insufficiency, or recurrent urinary tract infections. The risk reduction of signs of progression of BPH was 39% with doxazosin, 34% with finasteride, and 66% with combination therapy.

This study proved that the two classes of drugs used together were superior as compared with either type of drug alone; however, the practical issue is cost. Obviously, two drugs cost more than one. Therefore, in most cases, the physician will start treatment with one class of drug or the other and add the second drug only if the response to the first drug alone is not satisfactory.

JN: Because we're now learning that there have been thousands of long-term adverse reactions to drugs classified as COX-2 inhibitors, apart from the side effects of alpha blockers and 5 alpha reductase inhibitor drugs listed here, are there any serious (life-threatening) adverse reactions that have been recorded that patients have had from taking either or both of these drugs for a long period of time?

KL: No, these drugs are safe. There have been no life-threatening reactions.

39. What is the effect of 5 alpha reductase drugs on prostate cancer?

The final answer to that question has not been resolved. A recent study in the *New England Journal of Medicine* reports on almost 20,000 men 55 years of age or older with a normal digital rectal examination and a PSA level of less than 3.0 ng/ml who were treated with either finasteride or placebo for 7 years. At the end of the study, prostate cancer was diagnosed in 18.4% of the men in the finasteride group and 24.4% of the men in the placebo group. This difference was statistically significant.

It was also found in this study, however, that aggressive cancers (those with Gleason scores 7, 8, 9, or 10) were more common in the finasteride group than the placebo group. Specifically, of those men in the finasteride group who developed prostate cancer, 37% had these more aggressive cancers, whereas in the placebo group of those men who developed cancer, only 22.2% had these more aggressive tumors.

There is no easy explanation for these findings, and further studies are needed. Currently, a study, known as the REDUCE (The Reduction by Dutasteride of Prostate Cancer Events) trial, is underway to examine whether dutasteride, which blocks both type 1 and type 2 five alpha reductase, will reduce the incidence of prostate cancer. This study also examines whether the cancers that occur in those patients on dutasteride are of the more aggressive kind.

Currently, most urologists recommend the patient use 5 alpha reductase inhibitors to reduce BPH symptoms and not as anticancer agents.

40. What is the role of herbal therapy in BPH treatment?

This question is difficult to answer. Herbs are considered as food additives and not drugs and, as such, are not regulated by the Food and Drug Administration (FDA).

The production and marketing of herbs are essentially unregulated. Therefore, few randomized studies evaluate the efficacy of herbal therapy in the treatment of BPH.

41. Can saw palmetto be used to treat BPH?

Phytotherapy, or what is more commonly known as herbal therapy, has become increasingly popular in the treatment of BPH. About 30 herbal compounds have been used to treat prostatic urinary symptoms. The most popular of these is known as saw palmetto, which is the extract of the dried ripe fruit from the American dwarf saw palmetto plant, *Serenoa repens*.

Phytotherapy
the use of plants or plant extracts for medicinal purposes.

Until recently, the efficacy of saw palmetto was unknown. A recent study in the *New England Journal of Medicine* (2006;354:557–566), however, demonstrated that there was no significant difference between saw palmetto and placebo as measured by symptom scores or urinary flow rates. Unless subsequent reports refute this well-done study, it would seem that saw palmetto has no benefit in the treatment of BPH.

JN: However, because we do know that the substances that are part of saw palmetto, such as beta sitosterol, free fatty acids, and flavonoids, are also substances that have appeared in separate studies as possible prostate anticancer agents, have there been any studies to show whether any of these substances individually might be effective in working to inhibit growth of any prostate cells?

KL: Currently, no well-done studies show that herbal therapy reduces the risk of prostate cancer.

PART FIVE

Surgical Treatment of Benign Prostatic Hypertrophy

What is an open prostatectomy?

What are the side effects of surgical treatment of BPH?

What are the results of surgical treatment of BPH?

More …

42. What is an open prostatectomy?

Open prostatectomy

a technique to remove the prostate through a skin incision.

An **open prostatectomy** refers to the removal of the obstructing portion of a benign prostate through a surgical incision. Open prostatectomies are usually reserved for large prostates that weigh over 100 grams.

The most common approach to perform an open prostatectomy is through a lower abdominal incision that extends from the symphysis pubis to the umbilicus (belly button) (Figure 6).

After the surgeon enters the abdomen through this incision, he or she has two surgical choices. The first is to make an incision in the anterior (front) wall of the bladder to approach the prostate. This is called a

Suprapubic prostatectomy

removal of a portion of the prostate through a lower abdominal incision.

suprapubic prostatectomy. After the surgeon has entered the bladder, he or she can enucleate or shell out the center of the prostate with his or her index finger. After the inner portion of the prostate is enucleated, stitches are placed in the prostatic fossa (the shell of prostate that is left). Postoperatively, the patient is

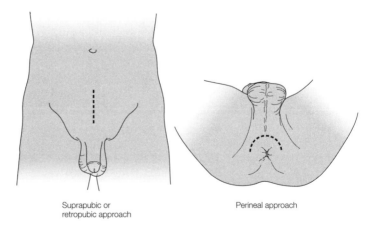

Suprapubic or
retropubic approach

Perineal approach

Figure 6   Types of surgical incisions for simple prostatectomy: suprapubic or retropubic approach and perineal approach.

left with a urethral catheter coming out of his penis and a suprapubic catheter coming out of the lower abdomen. A patient is usually in the hospital 3 or 4 days after a suprapubic prostatectomy.

A retropubic simple prostatectomy is similar to a suprapubic simple prostatectomy as it is also performed through a lower abdominal incision. When performing a retropubic simple prostatectomy, however, the urologist does not open the bladder but instead makes an incision through the prostate capsule. As is done with a suprapubic prostatectomy, the inner portion of the prostate is shelled out or enucleated. Because the bladder is not opened, it is not necessary to leave a suprapubic tube postoperatively, but a urethral catheter is left in place. Like a suprapubic simple prostatectomy, the patient is usually in the hospital 3 or 4 days postoperatively.

In addition to the abdominal approaches described previously here, a benign prostate can be surgically approached via the **perineum**. The perineum is the area between the scrotum and the anus. When this approach is used, the perineal skin incision is used to expose the prostate; then an incision is made in the prostatic capsule, and the prostate is enucleated, similar to a simple retropubic prostatectomy. A urethral catheter is left postoperatively, and the patient is usually in the hospital 1 to 2 days.

Perineum

in a male, the region between the scrotum and rectum.

43. What is a transurethral prostatectomy?

A **transurethral prostatectomy** (TURP) is an operation that is designed to remove the prostate through the urethra; no external incision is made. A TURP is

Transurethral prostatectomy

a method of removing obstructive prostate tissue through the urethra so that no external incision is made; also known as TURP.

Resectoscope

an instrument used
to remove (resect)
prostate, bladder, or
urethral tissue
through the urethra.

Hyponatremic

a low sodium level in
the blood.

**Transurethral
incision of the
prostate**

a method of remov-
ing prostatic obstruc-
tion using an incision
instead of resection;
also known as TUIP.

performed using a special instrument called a **resecto-scope**, which scrapes out the center of the prostate by using an electrical current that cuts out the tissue with a loop. In order to permit transmission of the electrical current from the loop to the tissue, the irrigating fluid normally used for a TURP is a glycine solution. This solution is somewhat more dilute than blood, and if the resection lasts a prolonged period of time, more than one hour, the patient can absorb too much fluid through the resected prostatic tissue bed and become **hyponatremic** (a low serum sodium). In severe cases, hyponatremia can cause neurologic symptoms, including seizures. Fortunately, these complications occur vary rarely. TURPs are usually limited to prostate glands of 100 grams or less.

After the TURP has been completed, a urethral catheter is left to enable irrigation of the bladder with fluid, typically for 1 to 2 days. After that period of time, the catheter is removed, and the patient is given a voiding trial.

JN: Can the Targis procedure be used on a patient who has had a TURP?

KL: Yes, it can.

44. What is a transurethral incision of the prostate?

A **transurethral incision of the prostate** (TUIP) is exactly that, an incision rather than a resection of the prostate. The technique of a TUIP is to use a special knife-like instrument called a Colling's knife that is placed through the same resectoscope sheath that is used for TURPs. Electrical current is transmitted through the knife, and two incisions are made at 5 o'clock and 7 o'clock through the bladder neck and prostate to the verumontanum where the ejaculatory ducts exit. The **verumontanum** is a landmark for the external sphincter, and the urologist does not want to cut beyond that. A depiction of a TUIP appears in Figures 7a and 7b.

Verumontanum
the area in the urethra where the ejaculatory ducts enter.

A TUIP as opposed to a TURP is a quicker, easier procedure. TUIPs tend to be used in younger men with smaller prostate glands. The incidence of retrograde ejaculation after TURP ranges from 50% to 95%, whereas the incidence is from 0% to 37% with TUIP. In properly selected patients, those with small glands, the rate of symptom relief with TUIP approaches that of TURP.

JN: If a man experiences problems with impotency after undergoing a TURP or TUIP, can those problems be corrected later?

KL: Postprostatectomy erectile dysfunction can be treated with a variety of medications or surgical implants.

45. What is electrovaporization of the prostate?

Electrovaporization of the prostate (TUVP) is, in a sense, a derivation of TURP. Rather than a resecting loop, the urologist uses a "roller ball" to heat and desiccate the prostate instead of actually resecting tissue (Figure 8).

Electrovaporization
a procedure in which electric current is used to destroy prostate tissue.

Electrovaporization of the prostate has been most often applied in patients with a history of bleeding disorders or in cases in which it is desired to minimize blood loss. Electrovaporization of the prostate tends to

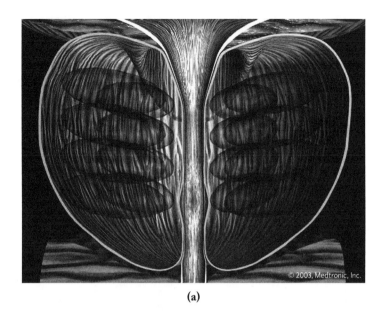

(a)

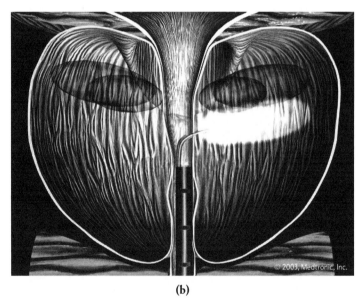

(b)

Figure 7   (a) Formation of lesions in the prostate. (b) Multiple lesions formed in the prostate. *Source:* **Courtesy of Medtronic, Inc. © Copyright 2003.**

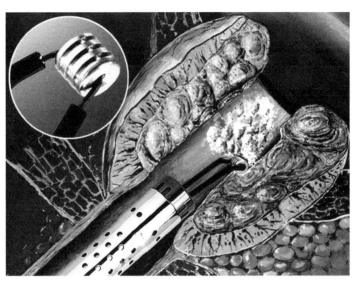

Figure 8   Electrovaporization of the prostate using a TURP VaporTrode®.
Source: **Courtesy of Gyrus ACMI, Southborough, MA.**

be used in patients with small- and medium-sized glands. Like TUIP, in properly selected patients, it is an alternative to TURP.

46. What are the side effects of surgical treatment of BPH?

The side effects associated with TURP can be divided into intraoperative and postoperative complications. A TURP is performed under either spinal or general anesthesia, and the usual complications that are associated with these forms of anesthesia can occur during a TURP. The introduction of either spinal or general anesthesia can result in hypotension or a drop in blood pressure.

Bleeding can occur with a TURP, and it is correlated with the size of the prostate and the duration of the operation; however, it should be emphasized that significant bleeding is uncommon when an experienced urologist performs the TURP.

Extravasation or perforation of the prostate can occur during a TURP. This causes some of the irrigation fluid used during a TURP to extravasate or leak outside the prostate. If the patient is awake under spinal anesthesia, this can result in nausea, vomiting, or abdominal pain. Most often, this complication can be managed by cessation of the operation and urethral catheter drainage. As with bleeding, extravasation in the hands of an experienced **resectionist** is uncommon.

The most dramatic complication that occurs intraoperatively or in the immediate postoperative period is the so-called TUR syndrome. In order to enable the urologist to see during a TURP, and for transmission of the electrical current, a somewhat dilute or hypotonic irrigation solution known as glycine is used during the TURP procedure. Variable amounts of the glycine are absorbed during a resection, depending on the amount of bleeding and length of time associated with the operation. Because of systemic absorption of relatively dilute fluid, some patients can develop a condition known as dilutional hyponatremia (low sodium) or the TUR syndrome. The manifestations of the TUR syndrome include nausea, vomiting, **brachycardia** or slow heart rate, and visual disturbances.

The treatment of the TUR syndrome is principally diuretic medications, which help the patient urinate out the excess fluid that has been absorbed. Some urologists will also give hypertonic saline or high-concentration sodium solutions to increase the serum

Extravasation

a discharge or escape of fluid, normally found in a vessel or tube, into the surrounding tissue.

Resectionist

the physician (urologist) who uses the resectoscope.

Brachycardia

a slow heart rate, usually under 60 beats per minute. A normal heart rate is from 60 to 100 beats per minute.

sodium. In most circumstances, the TUR syndrome can be corrected in the immediate postoperative period.

In the postoperative period, a very rare patient will continue to bleed after a TURP. The initial management is to replace the blood loss with appropriate blood transfusions and to increase the irrigation fluid that is used to irrigate the bladder through what is known as a three-way urethral catheter. Despite these maneuvers, some patients continue to bleed and require a return to the operating room to fulgurate (burn) the bleeding points present in the prostatic urethra.

47. What are the results of surgical treatment of BPH?

The TURP is a commonly done surgical procedure that urologists have performed for decades. It is a reliable method to relieve obstructive urinary symptoms. As mentioned previously here, complications associated with TURP can occur. Recent studies report that blood transfusions are required in about 4% of the patients who undergo the procedure. Because the apex of the prostate is near the external urinary sphincter, incontinence is a potential complication. Fortunately, the risk of urinary incontinence after a TURP has been estimated to be about 1%. Erectile dysfunction or impotence can occur after a TURP. It is theorized that some of the electrical current from the resectoscope loupe scatters beyond the prostate capsule and injures the nerves.

JN: Is there a way to preserve ejaculation after a TURP?

KL: There is a technique called "a bladder neck preserving TURP," which in some cases can preserve ejaculation after a TURP.

PART SIX

Minimally Invasive Surgery of Benign Prostatic Hypertrophy

What types of laser therapy are available?

What is microwave therapy of the prostate?

What other minimally invasive surgical treatments of the prostate are available?

More ...

48. What is minimally invasive surgical treatment of BPH?

Even though open prostatectomy and TURP, TUIP, and TUVP have been commonly performed, reliable operations, urologists have sought procedures that are less invasive and easier on the patients. These procedures have become known as minimally invasive surgical treatment (MIST) of BPH. These MIST techniques include laser procedures, hyperthermia and thermotherapy, radiofrequency ablation, balloon dilation of the prostate, urethral stents, and high-intensity focused ultrasound.

JN: If a man has a TURP, TUIP, or TUVP and finds that his prostate continues to enlarge even with two-medication therapy, is minimally invasive or other surgery now something that should be considered?

KL: Yes, these should be considered if medical therapy has failed.

49. What is laser therapy of the prostate?

Over the past 20 years, several generations of lasers have been used to treat obstructive prostate symptoms. LASER is an acronym for light-amplification stimulated emission resonance. In practical terms, this means that the light energy is very focused and allows powerful and precise application of the light energy to tissue.

The potential advantages of laser therapy include minimal bleeding, avoidance of TUR syndrome, less retrograde ejaculation, the ability to treat anticoagulated patients, and the potential to treat patients on an outpatient basis. We now review the various lasers that have been used to treat BPH.

50. What types of laser therapy are available?

Multiple types of lasers have been used throughout many areas of medical practice. In urology, several types of laser technology have been applied to the treatment of BPH. When considering whether laser therapy is appropriate for his prostate symptoms, it is important for the patient to have a thorough discussion with his urologist about the treatment options and which laser will be used and why. Not every urologist or every hospital has access to every laser that is on the market.

Lasers that are used for the treatment of an enlarged prostate have different characteristics. They have different methods of delivery, emit different wavelengths of light, and have variable tissue effects.

Several types of laser delivery systems have been used to treat prostate enlargement, including side-firing lasers, contact lasers, and interstitial lasers. In addition, lasers of variable wavelength have also been used in the treatment of BPH.

Laser applications to the treatment of BPH are still evolving, and no single laser type has gained preeminence. A new development in laser technology is the Green Light PVP laser. This laser has a wavelength of 532 nm and has a thermal coagulation depth of 1 to 2 mm. Early studies suggest that this laser in particular may be a very good option to a TURP. The Holmium:YAG laser is also emerging as an attractive laser alternative for the treatment of BPH. The Holmium:YAG laser operates in a pulsed mode in the near infrared area of the electromagnetic spectrum at a wavelength of 2140 nm. Its tissue absorption distance is 0.4 mm.

51. What are the results of laser therapy?

Many series reporting laser treatment of BPH suffer because they have no control group and have a short follow-up; however, laser therapy for BPH continues to generate interest because of two potential advantages: virtually no blood loss and the ability to perform laser surgery on an outpatient basis.

Laser technology continues to evolve rapidly, and not every hospital or urologist has access to every laser technology. The patient should discuss with the urologist what laser is to be used in his treatment and why, as well as what are the individual urologist's results.

52. What is microwave therapy of the prostate?

Microwave energy has been used to treat BPH using both transrectal and transurethral approaches, but most modern machines use the transurethral route. Current machines deliver microwave energy to the prostate via a transurethral catheter, and a transrectal balloon monitors rectal temperature simultaneously.

The treatment is delivered under local anesthesia on an outpatient basis and typically takes about one-half hour. The patient will go home with an indwelling urethral catheter for a period of days at the discretion of the urologist.

JN: Is a patient who has undergone microwave therapy for the prostate, now with a urethral catheter left in for 7 to 10 days, able to go about his business without much trouble? Should the catheter be removed by only a health care professional?

KL: Yes, the patient can generally go about his business without much trouble with a catheter in place. It is best to have the catheter removed by a health care professional.

53. What are the results of microwave therapy?

Results after microwave therapy can be grouped into two classes: subjective and objective. Subjective results use patient symptoms score sheets where the patients record their perception of their voiding characteristics. Objective results such as measurements of peak urinary flow rates and post void residual volumes are measured by the physician.

Using these criteria, several studies have shown improvement in both subjective and objective measurement following microwave therapy. This technology, however, is still relatively new, and long-term data are lacking. No one yet knows whether these promising early results are durable.

54. What is radiofrequency therapy of the prostate?

Radiofrequency treatment of BPH is commonly referred to as TUNA—transurethral needle ablation of the prostate. This technique involves placing interstitial radiofrequency needles through the urethra into the lateral prostatic lobes to cause coagulation necrosis.

The tissue is heated to 100°C at a radiofrequency power of 490 KHz for 4 minutes per lesion. The number of times the needles are placed into the prostatic lobes is at the discretion of the urologist based on the size of the prostate gland.

The TUNA device and generator are shown in Figures 9 and 10. Two needles that are at 60-degree angles to each other are deployed into the prostatic tissues by piercing the prostatic urethra. Each treatment with the needles treats prostate tissue about 1 cm in diameter.

55. What are the results of radiofrequency therapy?

TUNA of the prostate uses radiofrequency energy to treat the patient. As with most of the other MIST

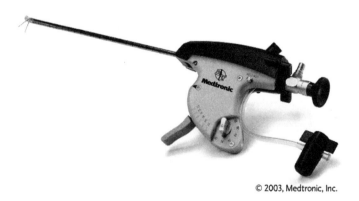

© 2003, Medtronic, Inc.

Figure 9 Precision™ Plus Hand Piece. *Source:* Courtesy of Medtronic, Inc. © Copyright 2003.

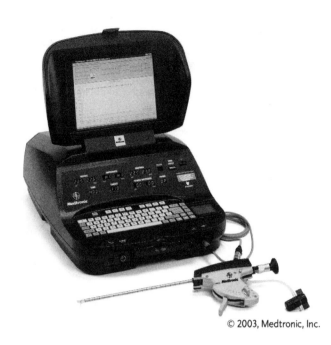

© 2003, Medtronic, Inc.

Figure 10   Precision™ Plus System (computer and hand piece). *Source:* Courtesy of Medtronic, Inc. © Copyright 2003.

results, few long-term data are available, and thus, results must be viewed with caution.

Table 4 contains combined TUNA results using both subjective and objective criteria.

56. What are prostatic stents?

Prostatic stents are devices that are placed transurethrally and expand to keep the prostatic urethra open. In many ways, they are similar to the coronary artery stents that have gained wide notoriety.

Prostatic stents
cylindrical devices that can be placed in the urethra to relieve prostatic obstruction.

Table 4 TUNA combined statistics

	Month Post Treatment	Number Patients	Preoperative	Postoperative	Percent Change
IPSS decrease	0	254	22		
Patient rerated	3	213		9	59
symptom scores	6	150		8	64
	12	29			
Qmax increase	0	254	8 ml/second		
Maximum	3	219		13	63
urinary flowrate	6	136		13	63
	12	35		14	75

The patients who are candidates for prostatic stents are fairly limited in number. Although some absorbable stents have been developed, they are not yet available for routine use. The clinically available stents are metallic and nonabsorbable. After they are placed, they are very difficult to remove.

Prostatic stents are most commonly used in older men who are in urinary retention requiring an indwelling urethral catheter and who are not candidates for any type of invasive therapy. After the stents have been in place for a few months, the mucosa or lining of the urethra grows through them, and they no longer can be seen cystoscopically.

57. What are the results of prostate stents?

As mentioned, in properly selected patients, prostatic stents can be very useful. The results of one specific type of prostatic stent called the UROLUME appear in Table 5.

Table 5 36-month follow-up North American Urolume study

	Month Post Treatment	Number Patients	Preoperative	Postoperative	Percent Change
Nonretention Cohort					
SS (Madsen) decrease	0	95	14		
Symptom score	36	95		5	65
Qmax increase	0	95	9 ml/second		
Maximum urinary flow rate	36	95		15	67
PVR decrease	0	95	89 ml		
Postroid residual	36	95		54	40
Retention Cohort					
SS (Madsen)	36	31	Retention	5	
Qmax	36	31	Retention	11 ml/second	
PVR	36	31	Retention	46 ml	

58. What is balloon dilation of the prostate?

In the late 1980s, balloon dilation of the prostate was introduced with great enthusiasm. The concept was similar to that of angioplasty of the coronary arteries, namely a balloon could dilate or stretch the prostatic urethra and thereby relieve obstruction. Several different types of balloons were developed and the early results were very encouraging.

Balloon dilation of the prostate was attractive because it could be done on an outpatient basis, although x-ray guidance of the balloon position and regional anesthesia were required.

59. What are the results of balloon dilation of the prostate?

Despite the encouraging early results, the improvement initially seen after balloon dilation of the prostate deteriorated over time. By about 2 years, several series showed that subjective and objective measurements had returned to baseline. Currently, balloon dilation of the prostate is no longer used and is considered obsolete.

60. What other minimally invasive surgical treatments of the prostate are available?

New ablative therapies of prostate tissue continue to be investigated. Among the most promising is alcohol injection of the prostate. This technology is still under development and is not clinically available except as a research protocol.

61. What is the role of a permanent indwelling urethral catheter in the treatment of BPH?

Some patients with prostatic obstruction and a weak bladder will not be able to void, regardless of what type of surgical intervention is employed. Some of these patients elect to be managed with an indwelling urethral catheter. The main drawback to an indwelling catheter is infection. In addition, sometimes the catheter can become plugged with blood or debris and needs to be changed emergently. Most patients with an indwelling urethral catheter have it changed by a visiting nurse at home or in the emergency room or their doctor's office at 1- to 2-month intervals.

An alternative to an indwelling urethral catheter is a **suprapubic tube**. A suprapubic tube can be placed percutaneously (through the skin) into the bladder through the lower abdominal wall. Many patients find a suprapubic tube more comfortable and easier to manage than a urethral catheter. Either the suprapubic tube or urethral catheter is connected to a drainage bag, which can be worn on the leg or hung on the side of bed. A suprapubic tube is typically changed by a nurse or physician as is the urethral catheter every 1 to 2 months.

62. What is the role of a clean intermittent catheterization in the treatment of BPH?

The problem with indwelling catheters is infection, as well as the fact that some patients find them cumbersome. If a patient is dexterous and motivated, he or she can be easily taught how to catheterize themselves every 4 to 6 hours.

This is a clean, but not sterile, procedure. Namely, the catheter should be clean but can be reused if necessary. Teenagers have been taught to do clean intermittent self-catheterization. It is not hard to do.

In circumstances in which a patient is unwilling or unable to perform self-catheterization, a family member can be taught how to perform the task.

63. What is the role of urecholine in the treatment of BPH?

Suprapubic tube

a type of catheter placed percutaneously (through the skin) into the bladder through the lower abdominal wall in order to drain urine.

Minimally Invasive Surgery of Benign Prostatic Hypertrophy

It is not uncommon for older men to go into urinary retention after any type of surgery that requires an anesthetic. Often these men are given a drug called urecholine that has been shown in laboratory studies in animals to stimulate bladder contractions.

The doses that can be used in humans, however, are pharmacologically inadequate to cause significant bladder contractions. Therefore, urecholine has little clinical value and should not be used in patients with urinary retention.

PART SEVEN

Prostatitis

What is prostatitis?

What types of prostatitis are there?

What is prostadynia?

More . . .

64. What is prostatitis?

Prostatitis refers to an inflammation of the prostate gland that can be manifested in a variety of ways. Symptoms of prostatitis include urinary frequency, urgency dysuria or painful urination, nocturia, perineal pain, low back pain, fever, and/or chills.

Prostatitis normally does not occur in children or adolescents, but can occur in adult men of any age. The diagnosis can be elusive and treatment is often empiric.

65. What types of prostatitis are there?

Prostatitis is generally divided into three general classifications: (1) acute and chronic bacterial prostatitis, (2) nonbacterial prostatitis, and (3) **prostadynia**.

Prostadynia

a spasm of the prostate that can cause symptoms similar to prostatitis.

Acute bacterial prostatitis is usually a sudden illness with irritative urinary symptoms and can be associated with fever. Urinary and/or prostatic secretions are often positive for bacteria. Some patients with acute prostatitis will have a transient elevation of their PSA. A PSA should not be done during an episode of acute prostatitis. If a PSA is inadvertently drawn during an episode of acute prostatitis and comes back elevated, a repeat PSA should be obtained after a course of antibiotics has been administered. Chronic bacterial prostatitis tends to be a more indolent condition. Irritative urinary symptoms are typical; however, fever is rare, and positive cultures are uncommon.

66. What is prostadynia?

Prostadynia has symptoms that are indistinguishable from prostatitis. A generation ago prostadynia was essentially considered the same as nonbacterial prostatitis; however, today, most urologists agree that prostadynia is caused by a spasm of the bladder neck, prostatic capsule, or prostatic urethra, whereas nonbacterial prostatitis may be caused by *Chlamydia trachomatis* or similar infectious agents.

67. How is prostatitis diagnosed?

The classic diagnostic maneuver for bacterial prostatitis is the so-called three-glass test. The patient is asked to void and collect his first 10 ml of urine. This is sent for culture and is known as VB1. Then the patient is asked to collect a midstream urine sample after he voids about 200 ml. This urine sample is sent for culture and is known as VB2. Then the urologist performs a digital rectal exam and massages the patient's prostate in an attempt to express prostatic secretions (EPS) into a sterile container. A prostatic massage is not always successful in producing sufficient secretions, and for some men, it can be quite uncomfortable. After the prostatic massage, the patient is asked to void again into a container, referred to as VB3, and this sample is sent for culture. If there is an increase in the number of bacterial colonies seen in either EPS or VB3, a diagnosis of bacterial prostatitis is made, and treatment is based on the antibiotic sensitivities of the organisms that were isolated.

68. How is prostatitis treated?

For most urologists, antibiotics are the first line of treatment for suspected prostatitis; however, the patient should recognize that if the urologist uses the three-glass test, many cases of prostatitis are treated empirically. In most cases of clinical prostatitis, a bacterial organism is not isolated. The urologist usually chooses an antibiotic that has pharmacokinetic properties that include good penetration into prostate tissue. Commonly used antibiotics for prostatitis include the sulfonamides and quinolones; however, the duration of time of antibiotic therapy also depends on the judgment of the urologist. It can vary from a week to months.

Because much of the treatment of clinical prostatitis is empiric, if a patient does not respond to the initial antibiotic treatment, the urologist will often switch the patient to a different antibiotic and then monitor the patient's clinical response.

Because the entity of nonbacterial prostatitis is also recognized and is often felt to be due to *Chlamydia trachomatis*, some urologists will give the patient a course of doxycycline, an antibiotic that covers Chlamydia particularly well.

69. How is prostadynia diagnosed?

Prostadynia is essentially a diagnosis of exclusion. If a patient is diagnosed with prostatitis, he will normally be treated with a course of antibiotics. If he does not respond clinically to the antibiotic, the urologist will usually either try another antibiotic or consider that the patient may have prostadynia. No objective clinical test or measurement is available that can be used to confirm a diagnosis of prostadynia. It is a clinical diagnosis made by the judgment of the treating urologist.

70. How is prostadynia treated?

Because prostadynia is felt to be due to a spasm or increased neurologic tone of the prostate, the class of drugs known as alpha blockers is used to treat prostadynia. Alpha blockers are the same group of drugs that can be used to treat signs of prostatic obstruction in patients with BPH.

The urologist will use the clinical response of the patient to alpha blockers to determine the length of time to continue treatment. Several alpha blockers are available, but no single drug in this class has been shown to be superior to the others in the treatment of prostadynia.

PART EIGHT

Prostate Cancer: Overview

How is prostate cancer diagnosed?

Is prostate cancer genetic?

Does nutrition influence prostate cancer?

More ...

71. Who gets prostate cancer?

Prostate cancer is a disease of middle-aged and older men. In 2005 it is estimated that there will be 232,090 new cases of prostate cancer diagnosed, and 30,350 men will die from prostate cancer. It has been estimated that one in eight white American men will develop prostate cancer in their lifetimes.

The difference in prostate cancer rates differs markedly by race. The incidence of prostate cancer in African Americans approaches 90 per 100,000 per year, in Caucasians 40 to 60 per 100,000 per year, and in Asians 2 to 10 per 100,000 per year. Asian men who move to the United States at a young age have higher rates than Asian men who remain in their native environment. This suggests that dietary and environmental factors may influence the rates of prostate cancer as well.

Family history also plays a significant role in the development of prostate cancer. It is estimated that a man with a first-degree relative with prostate cancer has a 2.1- to 2.8-fold greater risk of developing prostate cancer than the general population.

Diet also likely is important in prostate cancer development. High dietary fat content appears to confer a 1.6 to 1.9 times greater risk of prostate cancer development.

There has been controversy in the literature as to whether smoking history, occupation, or socioeconomic status is linked to prostate cancer. To date, there is no conclusive evidence that any of these factors significantly impacts the risk of prostate cancer.

JN: Scientists have been learning more about the role of inflammation as a marker for various diseases. Is there any reason to believe that there are toxic agents that might cause a prostate to become inflamed and that this inflammation might cause an infection that would start the process of creating prostate cancer cells?

KL: The answer to this question is not known. Researchers are looking into the link between prostate infection and prostate cancer.

72. How is prostate cancer diagnosed?

Prostate cancer is diagnosed by a digital rectal exam and a PSA blood test. It has been shown that a digital rectal exam and PSA test together are superior to either examination alone. Controversy exists, however, among regulatory bodies whether men should be screened for prostate cancer. Table 6 summarizes organizational policies on prostate cancer screening.

Those agencies that do endorse prostate cancer screening recommend that all men obtain an annual PSA test and digital rectal exam starting at the age of 50 years and those in high-risk groups, African American

Table 6 Organizational policies on prostate cancer screening

Organization	Policy on Prostate Cancer Screening
American Urologic Association	Pro
American Cancer Society	Pro
Food and Drug Administration	Pro
American Medical Association	Con
American College of Physicians	Con
United States Preventive Services Task Force	Con
European Union	Con

men, or with a family history start getting PSAs and digital rectal exams at the age of 40 years.

73. What is prostate ultrasound and biopsy?

A prostate ultrasound and biopsy is performed to obtain prostatic tissue to make a definitive diagnosis of prostate cancer. Without a tissue diagnosis, one cannot be sure that an individual man has prostate cancer regardless of his rectal exam or PSA level.

A prostate ultrasound and biopsy is usually done in the urologist's office. A patient typically will be asked to take antibiotics either before or after the biopsy depending on the individual urologist's custom. Many urologists also ask the patient to refrain from aspirin for 10 days before the biopsy to minimize the risk of bleeding and to administer a Fleet enema to himself the night before or morning of the biopsy to clean out the rectum.

The urologist may perform the ultrasound and biopsy by himself or with a radiologist or ultrasound technician. The patient is asked to lie on his side with his knees pulled up to his chest. Lubrication is placed in the rectum and an ultrasound probe, which is a plastic tube about the width of two fingers, is then placed in the rectum. This ultrasound probe transmits a picture of the prostate on to a screen where it is viewed by the urologist. Many urologists will then inject a local anesthetic into the surface of the prostate to numb the prostate before the biopsies are taken.

At this point, a spring-loaded biopsy gun is placed through a channel in the ultrasound probe. The biopsy gun takes small cores of tissue from the prostate. The number of cores taken is variable and depends on the judgment of the urologist. The prostate cores are sent to pathology for review and diagnosis. The typical ultrasound and prostate biopsies take 20 to 30 minutes. The patient is sent home on oral antibiotics, and the patient may see blood in his urine, stool, or semen for several days or at times for several weeks after the biopsies.

JN: Do negative results of a needle biopsy mean that the patient's prostate is free of cancer or that just the portions of the prostate that were selected for biopsy were free of cancer or that the cancer was so small that the biopsy made it difficult to identify?

KL: A negative biopsy does not categorically prove that the patient does not have cancer. Sampling error can occur and small tumors can be missed. Therefore, follow-up after a negative biopsy is important.

74. What are Gleason grades and scores?

For many years, pathologists described the histologic (microscopic) features of prostate cancer in a very imprecise way. Pathologists generally lumped prostate cancer into one of three categories: well, moderately, or poorly differentiated tumors. Then, in 1974, Donald Gleason, a pathologist at the University of Minnesota, published a set of reproducible criteria that pathologists could use to describe or grade prostate cancer. The grades ranged from 1 through 5, with 1 being the best or least aggressive cancer and 5 being the worst or most aggressive cancer. A Gleason score is calculated by adding together the two most prevalent grades in the tissue that the pathologist examines. Therefore, the best Gleason score is a $1 + 1 = 2$, and the worst is a $5 + 5 = 10$.

If the tumor is not homogenous, then the most prevalent grade is listed first, such as 5 + 4 = 9. It should be emphasized that a Gleason score 4 + 3 = 7 is different than a 3 + 4 = 7 because the most prevalent grade is higher. Almost all pathologists who examine prostate cancer now use the Gleason scoring system.

75. Is prostate cancer genetic?

To some degree prostate cancer is genetic. Prostate cancer rates differ significantly among racial and ethnic groups. African American men have an incidence of prostate cancer about 150/100,000 person-years. Caucasian men have an incidence at about 100/100,000 person-years, and Asian men have an incidence of about 30 to 40/100,000 person-years.

Family history is an important factor in determining whether a man is at an increased risk for prostate cancer. The more family members and the earlier the age of onset of the cancer in related family members increase the risk. Table 7 is from Carter et al. (*J Urol* 1993;150:797) and displays this relationship.

Table 7   Estimated risk ratios for prostate cancer in first-degree relatives of probands, by age at onset in proband (patients) and additional affected family members.

Age at Onset of Proband	Risk Ratio	
	No Additional Relative Affected	1 or More Additional First-Degree Relatives Affected
50	1.9 (1.2–2.8)	7.1 (3.7–13.6)
60	1.4 (1.1–1.7)	5.2 (3.1–8.7)
70	1.0[*]	3.8 (2.4–6.0)

[*]Reference group. Hazard ratio is shown with 95% confidence interval in parentheses.

Source: Carter BS, Bova GS, Beaty TH, et al. Hereditary prostate cancer: epidemiologic and clinical features. *J Urol.* 1993;150(3):797–802.

JN: If among men whose fathers had prostate cancer 55% of them also developed prostate cancer, is it scientifically reasonable to conclude that a principal factor in the case of the sons who developed cancer was genetic? If so, do we have any studies that suggest why 45% of the sons who didn't develop prostate cancer escaped the disease?

KL: We do not entirely understand the genetic influence of prostate cancer and its specific influence in an individual cancer.

*JN: What about **gene therapy** for prostate cancer?*

KL: Gene therapy is receiving much attention as a potential treatment for many cancers. Currently, gene therapy is still an experimental strategy for prostate cancer treatment.

Gene therapy
a technique used to correct defective genes.

76. How is prostate cancer staged?

The stage of a prostate cancer refers to the extent of the prostate, whether it is small and confined to the prostatic or whether it is metastatic and spread to other areas of the body.

Prostate cancer typically spreads locally through the prostate capsule and then to the regional lymph nodes known as the obturator and iliac nodes. Distant spread of prostate cancer typically goes to the bone or lungs.

Urologists commonly use two staging systems of prostate cancer. The older classification system is known as the Whitmore-Jewett classification and goes from A through D. The newer and more widely used system is the TNM classification, where T refers to the primary tumor, N to the regional lymph nodes, and M to metastases. Two staging systems appear in Table 8.

Table 8 Prostate cancer staging systems

TNM	Description	Whitmore-Jewett	Description
TX	Primary tumor cannot be assessed	None[*]	None
T0	No evidence of primary tumor	None	None
T1	Clinically unapparent tumor—not palpable or visible by imaging	A	Same as TNM
T1a	Tumor found incidentally in tissue removed at TUR; 5% or less of tissue is cancerous	A1	Same as TNM
T1b	Tumor found incidentally at TUR; more than 5% of tissue is cancerous	A2	Same as TNM
T1c	Tumor identified by prostate needle biopsy because of PSA elevation	None	None
T2	Palpable tumor confined within the prostate	B	Same as TNM
T2a	Tumor involves half of a lobe or less	B1N	Tumor involves half of a lobe or less; surrounded by normal tissue
T2b	Tumor involves more than half of a lobe, but not both lobes	B1	Tumor involves less than one lobe
T2c	Tumor involves both lobes	B2	Tumor involves one entire lobe or more
T3	Palpable tumor extending through prostate capsule and/or involving seminal vesicle(s)	C1	Tumor < 6 cm in diameter
T3a	Unilateral extracapsular extension	C1	Same as TNM
T3b	Bilateral extracapsular extension	C1	Same as TNM
T3c	Tumor invades seminal vesicle(s)	C1	Same as TNM

(*continued*)

Table 8 **(continued)**

TNM	Description	Whitmore-Jewett	Description
T4	Tumor is fixed or invades adjacent structures other than seminal vesicles	C2	Tumor < 6 cm in diameter
T4a	Tumor invades bladder neck and/or external sphincter and/or rectum	C2	Same as TNM
T4b	Tumor invades levator muscle and/or is fixed to pelvic wall	C2	Same as TNM
N+	Involvement of regional lymph nodes	D1	Same as TNM
None	None	D0	Elevation of prostatic acid phosphatase only (enzymatic assay)
NX	Regional lymph nodes cannot be assessed	None	None
N0	No regional lymph node metastasis	None	None
N1	Metastasis in a single regional lymph node, ≤ 2 cm in greatest dimension	D1	Same as TNM
N2	Metastasis in a single regional lymph node, > 2 cm but not > 5 cm in greatest dimension, or multiple regional lymph nodes, none > 5 cm in greatest dimension	D1	Same as TNM
N3	Metastasis in a regional lymph node > 5 cm in greatest dimension	D1	Same as TNM
M+	Distant metastatic spread	D2	Same as TNM

(continued)

Table 8   (continued)

TNM	Description	Whitmore-Jewett	Description
MX	Presence of distant metastases cannot be assessed	None	None
M0	No distant metastases	None	None
M1	Distant metastases	D2	Same as TNM
M1a	Involvement of nonregional lymph nodes	D2	Same as TNM
M1b	Involvement of bone(s)	D2	Same as TNM
M1c	Involvement of other distant sites	D2	Same as TNM
None	None	D3	Hormone refractory disease

*None = No comparable category

TUR, Transurethral resection; PSA, prostate-specific antigen.

77. Does nutrition influence prostate cancer?

Nutrition does influence prostate cancer, and there is still much about the relationship between nutrition and prostate cancer that we do not fully understand.

Dietary fat intake appears to be an important factor in influencing the development of prostate cancer. It has been postulated that high fat intake alters the production of sex hormones and thereby can alter the risk of prostate cancer.

Epidemiologic studies have shown that geographic areas with high fat content in the diet have higher death rates from prostate cancer. Japanese men have much lower fat content in their diets and much lower prostate cancer rates than U.S. men; however, Japanese men who move to the United States and adopt the higher fat content of Western diets have prostate cancer rates that are intermediate between the low risk in Japan and the higher risk in the United States.

Free radical scavengers that bind unpaired electrons in oxygen atoms have also been shown to be beneficial in preventing prostate cancer. Lycopenes are natural occurring free radical scavengers that are found in tomatoes and tomato products. Vitamin E and selenium have also been reported to lower the risk of developing prostate cancer.

Free radical scavengers

substances that can bind an atom or molecule with an unpaired electron.

JN: Some time ago a British medical journal (The Lancet 2001;358:641–642) reported that men with greater exposure to sunlight appear to have a reduced risk of prostate cancer. The actual number of men with lowest lifetime exposure to ultraviolet radiation had a three-fold greater risk of prostate cancer than did men with the highest life-time exposure. The assumed principal benefit of sunlight, in this case, was in the production of vitamin D. The study found that physiologic concentrations of the active from of vitamin D change the makeup of prostate cancer cells so that they are less likely to spread. The risk, of course, is that too much sunlight can cause skin cancer.

KL: There is evidence that exposure to sunlight and vita-min D production may have a beneficial effect in prevent-ing prostate cancer.

PART NINE

Prostate Cancer: Treatment for Localized Disease

What is a radical prostatectomy?

What is external beam radiation therapy?

What is cryotherapy?

More ...

78. What is observation only?

Observation only or watchful waiting refers to the approach of not instituting any therapy in a man with prostate cancer. The rationale for this strategy is that some older men who die from unrelated causes are found to have prostate cancer on autopsy. Such men are said to die with but not from the prostate cancer. This finding implies that some prostate cancers are indolent and do not need to be treated. The challenge is that there is no fool-proof way—not PSA level, Gleason score, or prostate cancer volume—to prove in an individual case whether the cancer is biologically indolent.

79. Who is a candidate for observation only?

Because the natural history of an individual prostate cancer is unknown, it is felt that older men with concomitant medical problems are the best candidates for observation only. In addition, it is wise to select tumors with low Gleason scores (6 or less) and low PSA levels (10 or less) and tumors that appear to be of a low volume. Even though no tumor characteristics guarantee an indolent course, the features of low Gleason score, low PSA, and low tumor volume are prognostic features that are often used to select patients for watchful waiting.

80. What are the results of observation only?

Several studies have been published on patients with prostate cancer who chose observation only or watchful waiting. The failure rates are higher than one might expect. In a report using the Connecticut Tumor Registry, it was found that death from prostate cancer at 15 years after diagnosis occurred in 9% of men with Gleason 2 to 4 score tumors, 28% of men with Gleason 5 to 7 score tumors, and 51% of men with Gleason 8 to 10 score tumors. It was estimated that the maximum lost life expectancy was 4 to 5 years in men with Gleason 5 to 7 tumors and 6 to 8 years in men with Gleason 8 to 10 tumors. These data would suggest that the best candidates for watchful waiting are men with a relatively short life expectancy and low Gleason score tumors. Patients who elect watchful waiting are generally followed with a PSA and digital rectal exam every 3 to 6 months.

81. What is a radical prostatectomy?

A **radical prostatectomy** refers to removing the entire prostate as opposed to a simple prostatectomy, which removes only the obstructing portion of the prostate. One way to think of it is in terms of an apple. A radical prostatectomy removes the core, the pulp, and the skin—the entire apple—whereas a simple prostatectomy removed the core and some of the surrounding pulp and leaves the outer pulp and the apple skin behind.

Radical prostatectomy
the surgical removal of the entire prostate and some of the surrounding tissue, done to treat prostate cancer.

A radical prostatectomy is performed for cancer cure. A simple prostatectomy is performed to relieve prostatic obstruction.

JN: Has removal of the prostate by laparoscopic surgery today become so successful a procedure that the risks of incontinence and impotence have been greatly reduced?

KL: No, currently, no single anatomic approach to a radical prostatectomy has proven superior to the others.

82. What types of radical prostatectomy are available?

Basically, three types of radical prostatectomy, which all accomplish the same thing (removal of the prostate), are available. The most commonly performed by urologists is the radical retropubic prostatectomy, which is performed through an incision in the lower abdomen. This approach enables the urologist to remove the pelvic lymph nodes, which drain the prostate and sometimes harbor cancer cells, at the same time as the radical prostatectomy.

A second approach is the laparoscopic radical prostatectomy. A laparoscopic radical prostatectomy is performed through a series of ports, which are small openings in the abdominal wall (between 5 to 12 mm), through which instruments are passed that can enable the urologist to perform a radical prostatectomy. The placement of the port sites can vary depending on the individual surgeon's preference, but a common configuration appears in Figure 11.

During a standard laparoscopic radical prostatectomy, the surgeon's hands directly control the laparoscopic instruments, but during a robotic prostatectomy, which also uses laparoscopic instruments, the surgeon sits at a console and controls the instrument through robotic arms. The lymph nodes that drain the prostate can be removed laparoscopically as well.

A final approach to a radical prostatectomy is the perineal prostatectomy, which is performed through the perineum, which is the skin between the scrotum and anus. The incision is small and the prostate is removed from below. The lymph nodes, however, cannot be

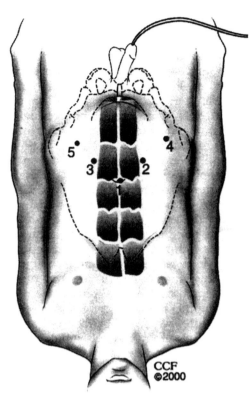

Figure 11 Laparoscopic radical prostatectomy port sites. *Source:* Reprinted with permission from *Urologic Clinics of North America*, Volume 28, Number 2, May 2001, p. 424. © WB Saunders Company.

removed through this incision as they can with the other techniques described. Therefore, if the surgeon feels that removing the lymph nodes is appropriate, he or she must remove them separately either laparoscopically or via a retropubic incision.

Much debate continues among urologists as to which surgical approach is best. There is no convincing evidence that any approach is intrinsically superior to the others. Much depends on the surgeon's personal experience. A patient considering undergoing a radical prostatectomy should have a thorough discussion with his surgeon about what surgical technique is to be used.

83. What are the potential side effects of a radical prostatectomy?

The two most common side effects of a radical prostatectomy are erectile dysfunction and urinary incontinence. Reported erectile dysfunction rates vary widely. This is due to some degree as to the method of reporting (whether the surgeon or some other party is conducting the questions) as well as how impotence is defined. Some authors consider the patient potent if he can achieve erections postoperatively with medication even though he did not require the medications preoperatively. Other factors that are important in preserving potency are the patient's age and size of tumor. Younger patients with smaller tumors have higher potency rates than older patients with larger tumors.

Urinary incontinence can also occur after any type of radical prostatectomy. Again, reported urinary incontinence rates vary depending on the method of reporting (surgeon interview versus blinded questionnaires) and definitions. Many patients experience improvement of urinary incontinence with time after surgery.

Other complications that can occur during or after a radical prostatectomy include bleeding, wound infection, ureteral injury, rectal injury, myocardial infarction, pulmonary embolus, prolonged urine leak, and thrombophlebitis. These complications are not common but can occur.

All patients considering having a radical prostatectomy should have a thorough discussion regarding potential complications and outcomes with their surgeon.

84. What are the results of radical prostatectomy?

A radical prostatectomy in properly selected patients offers the best chance for cure of prostate cancer. Patients with low stage, T1–T2 disease, and low Gleason scores of 6 or less, and a low preoperative PSA of 10 ng/dl or less can expect cure rates approaching 90% (Table 9).

85. What is external beam radiation therapy?

Radiation therapy of several types can cure some prostate cancers. External beam radiation therapy is typically given over a 6- to 7-week period. The patient comes into the hospital on a daily basis from Monday through Friday and is placed in a radiation therapy machine, where the radiation beam is focused on the prostate. Historically, the typical dose delivered to localized prostate cancer was in the 6,500- to 7,000-cGy range.

The total dose administered and the field of the radiation therapy depend on the grade and stage of the prostate cancer. Radiation therapy fields can be extended to include the pelvic lymph nodes if there is clinical suspicion or pathologic confirmation that they are positive for tumor.

Radiation therapy
radiation energy used to treat many types of cancer, usually administered over 6 to 7 weeks.

86. What is conformational radiation therapy?

Three-dimensional or conformational radiation therapy was developed as it became evident that a radiation dose of 6,500 to 7,000 cGy did not cure all prostate cancers. Conformational radiation therapy makes use of advanced computed tomography (CT)

Table 9   Radical prostatectomy results

Acturial (PSA-Based) %-Year Nonprogression Rates (5) After Radical Prostatectomy For Clinical Stage T1-2NXMO Prostate Cancer According to Clinical Stage, Biopsy Gleason Score, Preoperative Serum Prostate-Specific Antigen, and Pathologic Stage

	Partin et al, 1993a	Catalona and Smith, 1994	Zincke et al, 1994	Baylor
No. of patients	894	925	3170	672
Clinical Stage				
T1a	100	89	85	91
T1b	91			
T1c	100	99	97	
T2a	87	85	81	85
T2b	71	74	71	
T2c	69	78		
Gleason Score				
2–4	98	91	93	92
5	92	89	80	86
6	85	85		
7	62	59		
8–10	46	74	60	57
Preoperative PSA				
0–4	92	95	93	
4.1–10.0	83	93	81	
10.1–20.0	56	71	74	
< 20.0	45			71
Pathologic Stage				
Organ confined	97	91	-	95
Extracapsular extension	-	-	-	81
Seminal vesicle invasion	47	-	-	40
Positive lymph node(s)	15	-	-	35

techniques, which permit three-dimensional recon-struction of the prostatic gland.

This technology allows the radiation therapy to be more precisely focused on the prostate gland with less radiation scatter to surrounding tissues. Studies using conformational radiation therapy have documented a 14% reduction in the amount of radiation received by the bladder and rectum when treating prostate cancer. This translates into two advantages. First, higher radiation doses can be administered to the prostate, increasing the chances for cure. Second, with less radiation scatter to adjacent organs, there are fewer side effects from conformational radiation therapy.

Intensity-modulated radiation therapy is a newer, more advanced form of three-dimensional conformational radiation therapy. Using intensity-modulated radiation therapy techniques, radiation oncologists can now deliver radiation doses exceeding 8,000 cGy in some patients.

87. What are the side effects of external beam radiation?

Side effects can occur due to external beam radiation whether it is traditional type or conformational radiation therapy. Common side effects include impotence as well as radiation cystitis (inflammation of the bladder) and radiation proctitis (inflammation of the rectum).

88. What are the results of external beam radiation?

The major determinants of the results of radiation therapy are patient selection and the cumulative dose of the radiation given. D'amico has divided pretreatment prostate cancer patients into low-, intermediate-, and high-risk groups. These groups were defined as follows: low-risk stage T1c, T2a, PSA level $\leq$ 10 ng/ml, Gleason score $\leq$ 6; intermediate-risk stage 2b or PSA level > 10 and $\leq$ 20 ng ml or Gleason score 7; and high-risk patients stage T2c or PSA

Table 10   Radiation therapy results

Dose Group	Prognostic	5-Year Biochemical Relapse-Free Survival (%)
low (64–70 Gray)	low risk	83
high (75–81 Gray)	low risk	95
low (63–70 Gray)	intermediate risk	55
high (75–81 Gray)	intermediate risk	78
low (64–70 Gray)	high risk	23
high (75–81)	high risk	53

level > 20 ng/ml or Gleason score ≥ 8. Using these definitions, the results for external beam radiation can be stratified as seen in Table 10, adapted from the work of Zelefsky et al. (*Int J Radiat Oncol Biol Phys.* 1998;41(3):491–500).

89. What is brachytherapy?

Brachytherapy therapy is the delivery of radiation energy by the use of radioactive seeds. These seeds are placed percutaneously, through the skin, in the perineum, which is the area between the scrotum and the rectum. Brachytherapy has the potential advantages of delivering a high dose of radiation to the prostate with relative sparing of the surrounding tissues.

The placement of the seeds is done with image guidance provided by either an ultrasound or a magnetic resonance imaging (MRI). It is usually performed jointly by a radiation therapist and urologist under anesthesia in the operating room. It is done on an outpatient basis.

Several types of radioactive seeds are available to serve as radiation sources. The most commonly used are iodine 125, which has a half-life of 60 days, or palladium 103, which has a half-life of 17 days. Palladium 103 delivers a higher radiation dose and is used more commonly in patients with a higher Gleason score.

In circumstances in which it is suspected that the tumor may be beyond the prostate, some radiation therapists will also use a "boost" of external beam radiation in addition to the radioactive seeds.

90. What are the side effects of brachytherapy?

Radiation cystitis and proctitis can occur after brachytherapy, although these complications are rare, 2% to 4%. Urinary symptoms are more common. Frequency and urgency can occur in 20% to 30% of patients, and a small percentage of patients, less than 10%, may require a transurethral resection of the prostate because of urinary retention. Impotence rates of 20% to 40% have been reported after brachytherapy.

91. What are the results of brachytherapy?

As has been mentioned previously with both surgery and external beam radiation, the underlying pathology plays a major role in predicting the outcome of brachytherapy in an individual patient. For most T_1 and T_2 prostate tumors, however, brachytherapy cure rates of 70% to 80% can be anticipated.

92. What is cryotherapy?

Cryotherapy
freezing the prostate as a cancer treatment.

Cryotherapy refers to the freezing of tissue. Cryotherapy has been used to treat various tumors throughout the body, including prostate cancer. Cryotherapy is delivered in a manner similar to brachytherapy, namely via the perineal route under regional or spinal anesthesia on an outpatient basis.

Several cryotherapy probes are placed under ultrasound guidance, and liquid nitrogen is circulated in the probes to rapidly cool the prostate to −180°C. An ice ball forms at the tip of each probe, and this is verified by the ultrasound monitoring. There is some evidence that a freeze–thaw–freeze–thaw cycle or double-freeze technique results in greater tumor destruction, and many urologists employ this treatment strategy. The probes are removed and, in most cases, an indwelling urethral catheter is left for a few days. Cryosurgery was initially used as salvage therapy for prostate cancer after radiation failures; however, it is gaining wider acceptance as a primary therapy for localized prostate cancer.

93. What are the side effects of cryosurgery?

Cryosurgery is associated with several complications. Urinary incontinence can occur in a small percentage of patients, and impotence has been reported as well. Perineal pain has also been associated with cryoablation of prostate cancer, but the most devastating potential complication is a prostate–rectal fistula, which is leaking of urine from the prostatic urethra through the rectum. Fistula formulation, however, is rare in the hands of experienced urologists.

94. What are the results of cryosurgery of the prostate?

Cryosurgery has evolved considerably in recent years. Urethral sloughing or necrosis, which was a problem in the early experience, has been dramatically reduced by the use of a urethral warming catheter. Only a few long-term reports have been published on the use of cryosurgery for localized prostate cancer, but there is accumulating data that cryosurgery is a viable alternative to brachytherapy in patients who either refuse radical prostatectomy or are felt to be poor surgical risks.

Encouraging results are now being reported with cryosurgery patients with clinically localized prostate cancer. Using a posttreatment PSA level of 1.0 ng/ml, 5-year biochemical cure rates of 71% to 89% have been reported.

Prostate cryotherapy has also been used as "salvage" therapy in men who have failed external beam radiation therapy. The incidence of negative postcryotherapy positive prostate biopsies has ranged from 63% to 97%. It is uncertain, however, whether a positive biopsy implies whether the cancer is biologically active.

PART TEN

Prostate Cancer: Treatment for Metastatic Disease

How is metastatic disease diagnosed?

What are GnRH agonists?

What is combination therapy?

More ...

95. How is metastatic disease diagnosed?

Metastatic disease should be distinguished from locally advanced disease. In the Whitmore-Jewett classification, it is stage D disease, and in the TNM classification, it is N1, N2, N3 or M1a, M1b, or M1c. From a practical standpoint, metastatic prostate cancer most commonly goes to the pelvic lymph nodes or bones.

Although a serum PSA above 10 ng/ml or a Gleason score of 8, 9, or 10 significantly increases the risk of metastatic disease, PSA and Gleason scores are fairly nonspecific determinants of metastatic disease. Most urologists today rely on radiographic information as the most reliable way to stage a patient with prostate cancer before initiating treatment.

CT and MRI have both been used to stage prostate cancer. From the literature, it would appear that an MRI is superior to a CT in detecting lymph node involvement. It has been demonstrated that an MRI is helpful if the prostate cancer has penetrated through the prostate capsule and extended locally. It is important to recognize that in order to determine local prostate cancer extension, an endorectal coil MRI rather than a transabdominal MRI should be performed.

A radionuclide bone scan is used to detect prostatic cancer metastases to the skeleton. A bone scan entails an intravenous injection of a radioactive isotope that is selectively taken up by metastases to the skeleton. After the patient is injected with the isotope, he is placed under a machine that scans his skeleton and the rest of his body for uptake of the radioisotopes. Old trauma to the skeleton, such as healed fractures, can sometimes cause false positive readings on the bone scan. It has been shown that patients with a serum PSA level of 10 ng/ml rarely, if ever, have bone metastases; thus, in such patients, a bone scan is rarely ordered.

96. What is an orchiectomy?

An **orchiectomy** refers to removal of the testicles. The type of orchiectomy that is performed for control of prostate cancer is referred to as a bilateral (both testicles) simple orchiectomy.

Orchiectomy

surgical removal of one or both testes.

A bilateral simple orchiectomy is performed under local, spinal, or general anesthesia, depending on the preferences of the patient and the urologist. It is performed as outpatient surgery, and the patient goes home the day of surgery. A simple orchiectomy should be distinguished from a radical orchiectomy, which is performed for cancer of the testicle. A radical orchiectomy is performed through an inguinal incision, and the testicle and spermatic cord are removed together.

The reason for performing a bilateral simple orchiectomy for metastatic prostate cancer is that prostate cancer needs testosterone to grow. By removing the testicle, you remove 98% to 99% of the circulating testosterone, and this will cause most prostate cancers to go into remission, although hormone therapy alone rarely cures prostate cancer.

After a man undergoes a bilateral simple orchiectomy, he will experience decreased libido or sex drive and erectile function. He will also have hot flashes much like a woman does when she goes through menopause. Many men also lose some muscle mass and physical strength. After an orchiectomy, men will experience, to varying degrees, osteoporosis or thinning of bones.

The osteoporosis, if it becomes a problem, can be treated with medication. Finally, it may be obvious, but should be stated that men who undergo a bilateral orchiectomy no longer produce sperm and can no longer father children.

97. What are GnRH agonists?

GnRH stands for **gonadotropin-releasing hormone**. GnRH is synonymous with LHRH or luteinizing hormone-releasing hormone. GnRH is released by the hypothalamus in the brain and acts on the pituitary gland to release luteinizing hormone, which then acts on the Leydig cells in the testicle to make testosterone. Circulating testosterone then stimulates prostate cancer growth.

GnRH agonists initially actually stimulate luteinizing hormone release by the pituitary and subsequent testosterone production by the testicle. Therefore, treatment initially causes a rise in testosterone levels for the first week or so of treatment. This can actually result in a "disease flare" or exacerbation of bone pain from bone metastases if they are present in the patient. This "disease flare" from the transient rise of serum testosterone after initiation of GnRH therapy can be blocked by the use of **antiandrogen** drugs, which bind to androgen receptors of cells in the body, thereby rendering the cells "blind" to the effects of testosterone. We speak more fully about antiandrogens in Question 98.

The reason that GnRH agonists work is that after about a week the GnRH agonists actually cause a downregulation of the receptors in the pituitary cells, which results in a decrease of LH production and subsequent testosterone levels.

Gonadotropin-releasing hormone

a hormone made by the hypothalamus that in turn stimulates the pituitary gland; abbreviated GnRH.

Antiandrogen

drugs that counteract the action of testosterone.

GnRH agonists have been around for more than 3 decades and are an accepted alternative to bilateral orchiectomy. Recently, however, a drug, Plenaxis, which is a GnRH antagonist, has been developed. When a GnRH antagonist such as Plenaxis is used, there is an immediate inhibition of luteinizing hormone and testosterone suppression. Therefore, there is no "disease flare" or need for use of antiandrogens.

Bilateral orchiectomy, GnRH agonists, and GnRH antagonists are all equivalent therapeutically. Which therapy to use is basically a lifestyle choice for the patient. A bilateral orchiectomy is done once and is permanent. Although a minor surgical procedure, however, it is still surgery, and some men psychologically don't like the idea of having their testicles removed.

GnRH agonists and antagonists have the same side effects as bilateral orchiectomy, such as decreased libido, erectile dysfunction, hot flashes, and loss of muscle mass, but avoid a surgical procedure. The GnRH agonists and antagonists are administered in the form of shots into the buttocks and come in varying doses so that the injections can be given every month, every 3 months, or once a year.

98. What are antiandrogens?

Antiandrogens are oral compounds that bind target cell androgen receptors, which prevent the uptake of testosterone. Antiandrogens are competitive inhibitors that prevent the binding of both DHT and testosterone to receptors in the cystoplasm of cells.

Two general classes of antiandrogens exist. The first type, steroidal antiandrogens, such as cyproterone acetate and megestrol acetate, are not commonly used in clinical practice any more. The second type, non-steroidal antiandrogens, such as eulexin (flutamide), nilutamide (nilandron), and bicalutamide (casodex), are much more commonly used clinically. Like any class of drugs, these drugs can have side effects that may include liver dysfunction, breast tenderness, breast enlargement (gynecomastia), and gastrointestinal side effects such as diarrhea, nausea, or vomiting. Sexual dysfunction is less common with the antiandrogens than with GnRH agonists or antagonists.

Today, antiandrogens are most commonly used with GnRH agonists. Some physicians, however, will treat patients with metastatic disease with antiandrogens as monotherapy or single agents.

Finally, the first antiandrogen drug that was ever used was estrogen. Estrogens are viewed as equivalent to testosterone from the point of view of the hypothalamus. Therefore, when a patient is given oral estrogens, the feedback "tricks" the hypothalamus into "thinking" that there is too much testosterone, and the hypothalamus responds by decreasing GnRH production, which subsequently decreases leuteinizing hormone and finally drops the serum testosterone.

Estrogen therapy, although relatively inexpensive, is rarely used today because of side effects. These side effects include loss of libido, sexual dysfunction, and decreased muscle mass, but more importantly, there are serious vascular side effects, which include deep venous thrombosis (blood clots in the legs) as well as strokes.

99. What is combination therapy?

Combination therapy refers to using a GnRH agonist or antagonist together with an antiandrogen. This results in what is known as total androgen blockade. This total androgen blockade is not transient, as is the case with the prevention of a "disease flare" after initiation of GnRH agonist therapy, but rather, combination therapy is often used on a permanent basis. The rationale behind this is the result of several studies that report that the use of combination therapy as compared with GnRH agonists or orchiectomy alone results in a slight survival advantage to the patient (see Table 11); however, not all physicians agree that combination therapy provides a significant advantage, and the patient should discuss these options thoroughly with his physician.

Table 11 Results of combination hormonal therapy

Study	No. Patients	Treatment	Median Time to Failure (mo)	Median Overall Survival (mo)
Crawford et al.	603	leuprolide	13.9*	28.3*
		leuprolide + flutamide 1	16.5*	35.6*
Denis et al.	327	orchiectomy	21.2*	28.8*
		goserelin + flutamide	44.2*	43.9*
Beland et al.	174	orchiectomy	11.7	18.9
		orchiectomy + nilutamide	12.4	24.3
Boccardo et al.	373	goserelin	12.0	32.0
		goserelin + flutamide	12.0	34.0

*Statistically significant

Goserelin = goserelin acetate

Source: Kantoff PW, Wishnow KI, Loughlin KR, eds. *Prostate Cancer: A Multidisciplinary Guide.* Cambridge, Mass: Blackwell Science; 1997:213.

100. What other therapy is available for metastatic disease?

Other options are available for the treatment of metastatic prostate cancer. If a patient has symptomatic or painful skeletal metastases, local radiation therapy can be useful.

Also other drugs such as corticosteroids, ketoconazole, and aminoglutethimide are oral agents that can be tried if standard hormone therapy has failed.

Chemotherapeutic drugs are also being used for patients who have developed hormone-refractory prostate cancer—namely patients who were initially on hormone therapy but whose prostate cancer has mutated, which permits it to grow even in the face of low testosterone levels.

A variety of chemotherapeutic drugs have been used in the treatment of hormone-refractory prostate cancer. Some of these agents include cisplatin, vinblastine, doxorubicin, and mitoxanthrone. Before considering whether to use chemotherapy and which specific drugs and doses should be considered, a patient should have a thorough discussion with a medical oncologist.

Supplements and the Prostate

The following nutrients, supplements, and substances have been the focus of many studies and individual reports on the effect that they might have on the prostate.

Supplements

Are they safe? What is the role of the FDA in connection with supplements? How does the Dietary Supplement and Health Education Act (DSHEA) affect supplements? Let's start with what is a dietary supplement. Traditionally, dietary supplements referred to products made of one or more of the essential nutrients, such as vitamins, minerals, and proteins, but DSHEA broadens the definition to include, with some exceptions, any products intended for ingestion as a supplement to the diet. This includes vitamins, minerals, herbs, botanicals, other plant-derived substances, amino acids (the individual building blocks of protein), concentrates, metabolite constituents, and extracts of these substances.

It's easy to spot a supplement because DSHEA requires manufacturers to include the words "dietary supplement" on product labels. Also, starting in March 1999, a "Supplemental Facts" panel is required on the labels of most dietary supplements.

The FDA oversees safety, manufacturing, and product information, such as claims in a product's labeling package inserts and accompanying literature. The Federal Trade Commission regulates the advertising of dietary supplements.

A product sold as a supplement and touted in its labeling as a new treatment or cure for a specific disease or condition would be considered unauthorized and illegal. Labeling changes consistent with the provisions in DSHEA would be required to maintain the product's status as a dietary supplement.

Meanwhile, remember that dietary supplements are not replacements for conventional diets. Supplements do not provide all of the known and perhaps unknown nutritional benefits of conventional food.

Monitoring for Safety

As with food, federal law requires manufacturers of dietary supplements to ensure that the products they put in the market are safe, but supplement manufacturers do not have to provide information to the FDA to get a product on the market, unlike the food additive process often required with new food ingredients. The FDA review and approval of supplement ingredients and products are not required before marketing, but manufacturers may not make certain claims about what the supplements can do.

Food additives that are not generally recognized as safe must undergo the FDA's premarket approval process for new food ingredients. This requires manufacturers to conduct safety studies and submit the results to the FDA for review before the ingredient can be used in marketed products. Based on its review, the FDA either authorizes or rejects the food additive.

Dietary supplement manufacturers that wish to market a new ingredient (i.e., an ingredient not marketed in the United States before 1994) have two options. The first involves submitting to the FDA at least 75 days before the product is expected to go on the market information that supports their conclusion that a new ingredient can reasonably be expected to be safe—"safe," meaning that the new ingredient does not present a significant or unreasonable risk of illness or injury under conditions of use recommended in the product's labeling.

Under DSHEA, after a dietary supplement is marketed, the FDA has the responsibility for showing that a dietary supplemental is unsafe before it can take action to restrict the product's use; however, the DSHEA prohibits supplement manufacturers from selling supplements that claim to diagnose, treat, prevent, or cure any disease.

Besides the FDA, individual states can take steps to restrict or stop the sale of potentially harmful dietary supplements within their jurisdiction. For example, Florida has banned some ephedra-containing products, and other states have said they are considering a similar action.

Under DSHEA and previous food labeling laws, supplement manufacturers are allowed to use documented claims on nutrient content and nutrition support claims, which include "structure-function claims."

Nutrient content claims describe the level of a nutrient in a food or dietary supplement. For example, a supplement containing at least 200 milligrams of calcium per serving could carry the claim "high in calcium." A supplement with at least 12 mg per serving of vitamin C could state on its label "Excellent source of vitamin C."

Nutrition

Support claims can describe a link between a nutrient and the deficiency disease that can result if the nutrient is lacking in the diet. For example, the label of a vitamin C supplement could state that vitamin C prevents scurvy. When these types of claims are used, the label must mention the prevalence of the nutrient deficiency disease in the United States.

These claims also refer to the supplement's effect on the body's structure or function, including its overall effect on a person's well-being. These are known as structure–function claims.

Examples of structure-function claims are as follows:

- Calcium builds strong bones.
- Antioxidants maintain cell integrity.
- Fiber maintains bowel regularity.

Fraudulent Products

In spite of the regulations designed to protect consumers, you need to be on the lookout for fraudulent products. These are products that don't do what they say they can or don't contain what they say they contain. At the very least, they waste consumers' money, and they may cause physical harm. For example:

1. Claims that the product is a "secret cure" and use of such terms as "breakthrough" "magical," "miracle cure," and "new discovery" are a warning. If the product were a cure for a serious disease, it would be widely reported in the media and used by health care professionals.

2. "Pseudomedical" jargon, such as "detoxify," "purify," and "energize," to describe a product's effects. These claims are vague and hard to measure, as are claims that the product can cure a wide range of unrelated diseases. No product can do that.

3. Claims that a product is backed by scientific studies, but with no list of references or references that are inadequate (i.e., if a list of references is provided, the citations cannot be traced, or if they are traceable, the studies are out of date, irrelevant, or poorly designed).

Quality Products

Poor manufacturing practices are not unique to dietary supplements, but the growing market for supplements in a less restrictive regulatory environment creates the potential for supplements to be prone to quality control problems. For example, the FDA has identified several problems in which some manufacturers were buying herbs, plants, and other ingredients without first adequately testing them to determine whether the product they ordered was actually what they received or whether the ingredients were free from contaminants.

Supplement users who suffer a serious harmful effect or illness that they think is related to supplement use should call a doctor or other healthcare provider. He or she in turn can report it to FDA MedWatch by calling 1-800-FDA-1088 or going to www.fda.gov/medwatch/report/hcp.htm on the MedWatch website. Patient names are kept confidential.

Consumers also may call the toll-free MedWatch number or go to www.fda.gov/medwatch/report/comsumer/consumer.htm on the MedWatch website to report an adverse reaction. To file a report, consumers will be asked to provide the following:

- Name, address, and telephone number of the person who became ill
- Name and address of the doctor or hospital providing medical treatment
- A description of the problem
- The name of the product and store. Report the problem to the manufacturer or distributor listed on the product's label and to the store where the product was bought.

Reading and Reporting

Consumers who use dietary supplements should always read product labels, follow directions, and heed all warnings.

Supplement Research Affecting the Prostate

A number of supplements have been studied for their possible effects on the prostate, and we have included brief summaries from the better known supplements here. The results of the studies should not be considered in any way as a recommendation of any supplement by the publisher. Moreover, these summaries do not include every published study or report of clinical trials.

Vitamin E: After years of almost universal acclaim for the importance and benefits of this vitamin, several disappointing studies have now been published. The disappointing results of an analysis of 19 studies, one of which found a "statistically significant risk" in vitamin E and three of which found no increased risk, caused one leading medical school to withdraw its recommendation for taking vitamin E.

At almost the same time, a major study of Finnish men revealed that vitamin E, with alpha- and gamma-tocopherols, appeared to cut the risk of prostate cancer by 50%. The numbers are the results from comparing 100 men with prostate cancer to 200 men without prostate cancer in a study known as the Alpha-Tocopherol, Beta Carotene Cancer Prevention Study, ultimately involving 30,000 Finnish men. The National Cancer Institute reported men with the highest levels of alpha-tocopherol were 51% less likely to develop prostate cancer, and men with the highest levels of gamma tocopherol were 43% less likely to develop prostate cancer.

What may have been overlooked in some of these studies of vitamin E is that a synthetic form of the vitamin, in which some of the oils have been extracted, may have been used. The natural form of vitamin E, as in the foods themselves, contains all four of the essential tocopherols—alpha, beta, gamma, and delta.

As for safety and value of vitamin E, the Institute of Medicine of the National Academy of Sciences believe that the safe upper limits for vitamin E is 1,500 IU a day, but the recommended daily allowances is only 23 IU or about 15 mg. Meanwhile, the position of the National Cancer Institute is that because oxidative stress is known to be a factor in prostate cancer, vitamin E, with its antioxidant activity, could be very important.

The bottom line on vitamin E is this: If you take the supplement, take one that has the natural vitamin E with all four tocopherols (available in most health stores), and follow the Institute of Medicine's recommended daily allowance of 15 mg. Nevertheless, try to get as much as you need from the foods you eat. To help with this, ask your doctor.

Selenium: This is a trace element. Low dietary intakes of it have been associated with prostate cancers. Selenium is also recognized for its immune-enhancing effects. The National

Cancer Institute is testing selenium alone and selenium in combination with vitamin E. One earlier study of 11,000 men revealed that selenium alone and vitamin E alone are less effective in preventing prostate cancer than are the two combined. Some research studies suggest that one reason those men with selenium deficiency are at risk is because inadequate levels of selenium let carcinogens multiply in the body. The U.S. recommended daily allowance for men over 50 years old is 70 micrograms. As with other supplements, too much selenium can be toxic. Selenium toxicity can cause hair and nail loss, rash, and fatigue.

Soy: Soybeans have high amounts of isoflavones, which contain phytochemicals believed to help prevent prostate and other cancers. Several studies suggest that foods containing soy isoflavones are associated with reduced incidence of some cancers, and the beneficial effects of taking soy appear to be immediate. In one study, as little as 2 ounces of soy grits a day, added to the diet of men with prostate cancer, produced a substantial reduction in PSA levels within 1 month.

Zinc: Although zinc is found in high concentrations in the prostate, which would seem to be a benefit, there are studies showing that men who took many times more than the recommended daily allowance (11 mg) of zinc for as long as 10 years (some men taking 100 mg or more daily for 10 years) were more than twice as likely to develop prostate cancer; however, excessive amounts of zinc may have quite different effects than those from using recommended daily amounts. A study conducted by the Chicago Medical School, in collaboration with researchers at the Cook County Hospital, on 5,000 patients indicated that zinc can prevent prostate enlargement. The National Cancer Institute's position on zinc is that although it is not clear how too much zinc may act to increase prostate cancer risk, until we do know, it would be wise to stay within the recommended daily allowance of 11 mg. Although we don't know how massive doses of zinc may act to increase prostate cancer risk, we do know that the immune system and the synthesis of DNA do require zinc.

Lycopene: This is one of the chemical substances that has appeared as a possible anticancer agent in dozens of studies. It is a member of the carotenoid family of substances and is found largely in tomatoes (especially in cooked tomatoes), tomato-based products, watermelon, and pink grapefruit. One study of lycopene showed that men who ate tomatoes at least two times a week had a lower risk of prostate cancer than those who did not. The study put the number at a 20% lower risk of prostate cancer for the men who ate stewed tomatoes twice a week. Other studies have shown major protective benefits of tomatoes and tomato-based products among men who ate five servings a week. In spite of the positive results from so many studies, some researchers caution that we should not conclude that it is the lycopene alone that produces the benefits, as there are other helpful substances in tomatoes that might help to protect against prostate cancer. Although we don't know everything about the actions of lycopene, we do know that it is one of the most powerful antioxidants that helps to neutralize oxidative stress and that although we don't know exactly why it is so good for our prostate health, we do know that eating more fruits and vegetables is good for our overall health.

Flaxseed: This appears to be one of the less well understood nutrients that might affect the prostate. One study involving several thousand men showed that the risk of prostate cancer among those who took alpha-linolenic acid was 70% higher than among men who didn't. Another small study showed the linolenic acid, which is a main component of flaxseed oil, lowered PSA from 8.5 to 5.7 in the men tested. A Duke University study showed that flaxseed was able to slow the growth of prostate tumors in mice, but the findings so far are insufficient to be able to say that flaxseed and flaxseed oil might be helpful in treating prostate problems.

Boron: The UCLA School of Public Health has compared the dietary patterns of 76 men with prostate cancer with that of 7,651 males without cancer. The greater the quantity of boron-rich foods consumed, the greater the reduction in the risk of being diagnosed with prostate cancer. Those men consuming the most boron (i.e., in the upper quartile of boron consumption) had a 64% reduction in prostate cancer, whereas men in the second quartile had a 35% reduction in risk and those in the third quartile reduced their risk by 24%. Men in the lowest quartile of boron consumption ate roughly one slice of fruit per day, whereas those in the highest quartile consumed 3.5 servings of fruit per day plus one serving of nuts. Boron-rich foods include plums, grapes, prunes, avocados, and nuts such as almonds and peanuts. A serving of 100 grams of prunes (12 dried prunes) has 2 to 3 mg of boron and 6.1 grams of fiber.

Summing Up: In discussing supplements, readers should be aware that well-known doctors and celebrities who have endorsed specific brands of supplements do receive substantial profits from the sale of the products they endorse. Receiving a profit from the sale of a supplement does not mean that the supplement is not as good as the endorser says; it does mean that the consumer should be aware of the endorser's financial interests in the supplement's success. Thus, make sure to ask your doctor about any supplements or herbal remedies that you are considering as an alternative treatment for the prostate. Your doctor will be able to tell you of the supplement's known actions and the mechanisms it uses to achieve its effects, such as absorption, metabolism, and excretion. Your doctor will also help you to evaluate the claims advanced for the different products and the possible interactions and reactions.

Support Groups

US TOO Group
Affiliation: Southeast Alabama Medical Center
Doctor's Building
SE Alabama Medical Center, 7th Floor
1108 Ross Clark Circle
Dothan, AL 36301
334-794-3216
Meets the first Thursday of each month at 7:00 PM

US TOO PC Survivor Support Group
389 Clubhouse Drive, #DD4
Gulf Shores, AL 36542
334-968-1115
Meets the first Thursday of each month, except September, and then on 9/21
Prostate Cancer Support Group
Affiliation: Fountain Valley Regional Hospital
11250 Warner Avenue
East Tower Cafeteria
Fountain Valley, CA
714-966-8055

Prostate Cancer Survivor's Support Group
200 Mowry Avenue at Civic Center Drive
Freemont, CA
Washington Hospital
510-657-0759
Meets each third Thursday, 7:00 to 9:00 PM, co-ed

The Prostate Forum, Fullerton
1st Presbyterian Church
838 N. Euclid, Fullerton, CA
714-607-9241
Meets the second Tuesday and the fourth Tuesday from 11 AM
    to 3 PM and 6 to 9 PM

Prostate Cancer Support Group
Medical Library at Marin General Hospital
Greenbrae on Bon Air Road
415-459-4668
Meets each Tuesday evening from 7:00 to 8:30 PM

Palo Alto VA Prostate Support Group
VA Palo Alto Health Care System
Building 101 Auditorium (1st floor near chapel)
408-996-7582
Meets the third Tuesday of every month from 11:00 AM to
    12:30 PM

Redwood City Support Group
702 Marshall Street
Redwood City, CA
650-367-5998
Meets on the first Tuesday of every month from 2:00 to 3:30 PM

San Jose Prostate Cancer Support Group
Camden Lifetime Activity Center
3369 Union Avenue (just North of Camden Avenue)
San Jose, CA
408-559-8553
Meets every second Wednesday of the month from 12:30 to
    2:30 PM

San Mateo Support Group
Mid-Peninsula Medical Arts Bldg.
1720 El Camino Real-Atrium Room, Burlingame
San Mateo, CA
650-572-9035
Meets on the third Thursday from 1 to 3 PM

Santa Barbara PC Support Group
Burntress Auditorium, Cancer Center of Santa Barbara
300 W. Pueblo
Santa Barbara, CA
806-682-7300 or 805-969-7166
Meets on the second and fourth Thursdays from 2:30 to 3:30 PM

**Santa Clara County: African American Prostate Cancer
   Support Group**
408-226-3947

Santa Cruz County Prostate Cancer Support Group
Affiliation: US TOO, ACS

Dominican Hospital, Katz Cancer Resource Center
Website: www.scprostate.org
831-724-6446
Meets on the last Tuesday of the month from 7 to 9 PM

UCSF Comprehensive Cancer Center
San Francisco, CA
415-885-3693
Meets on the second and fourth Wednesdays from 6 to 7 PM

Silicon Valley Prostate Cancer Support
2500 Grant Road, Mountain View
Basement of El Camino Hospital
Meets every first Thursday of the month from 7 to 9 PM

Simi Valley US TOO Prostate Cancer Support Group
Aspen Center
2750 Sycamore Drive, Simi Valley
Simi Valley, CA
805-522-4782

Jupiter Hospital
Jupiter, FL
561-743-5069
Meets every second Wednesday of every month at 5 PM

Man to Man
Auditorium of Sarasota Memorial Hospital
1700 S. Tamiami Trail (Rt. 41)
Sarasota, FL
941-378-5647
Meets every fourth Monday of month at 2 PM

Prostate Support Association
Affiliation: Emory Healthcare
Emory Clinic
1365 Clifton Road, B Building, 5th Floor Conference Room
Atlanta, GA
404-727-4328

Man to Man/Side by Side
Affiliation: American Cancer Society
Diversified Health Care Services
510 West Park
Champaign, IL
217-352-3042
Meets the first Thursday from 7:00 to 8:30 PM

Man to Man Education and Support Group
Affiliation: American Cancer Society, St. Vincent Hospital
Cooling Auditorium at St. Vincent Hospital
2001 W. 86th St.
Indianapolis, IN
317-849-1022
Meets from 6:45 to 8:30 PM

Well County Man to Man
Affiliation: American Cancer Society, Man to Man
Wells County Council on Aging
225 W. Water St.
Bluffton, IN 46714
260-824-2986
Meets every second Monday of each month from 4 to 5:30 PM

US TOO Chapter
Via Christi-St. Joseph Medical Center
East Campus
3600 E. Harry
Wichita, KS
316-943-8274
Meets every second Monday of each month

Robert D. Knepper Man to Man Group
Affiliation: America Cancer Society
May Bird Perkins Cancer Center
4950 Essen Lane
Baton Rouge, LA
Meets the first Monday of each month from 7 to 9 PM

Man to Man Worcester County
Atlantic General Health Center, Ocean Pines Offices
11107 Racetrack Road
Berlin, MD
410-208-9555
Meets the first Tuesday of each month from 7:00 to 8:30 PM

Suburban Hospital
Bethesda, MD
301-896-3939
Meets on the third Monday of the month from 7:00 to 8:30 PM
    in conference rooms 6 and 7

VFW Prostate Cancer Support Group of DelMarVa
821 E. William Street
Salisbury, MD
410-835-2850
Meets at VFW Post 194 on the second Tuesday of the month for
    lunch, 1:30 PM for meeting

The "Survivor's Association"
Grand Rapids, MI
616-356-4349
Meets at 7 PM on the first Tuesday of each month from
    September to June

Prostate Support Group
West Michigan Cancer Center
200 N. Park St.
Kalamazoo, MI
800-999-9748
Meets monthly on the last Wednesday at 7 PM

Appendix B

Prostate Cancer Support of Lee County
Affiliations: Man to Man, US TOO
Enrichment Center
1615 South Third Street
Sanford, NC 27330
919-774-6685
Meets on the second Wednesday of the month from 11:00 to
  12:30 PM

**Prostate Cancer Support Association of New Mexico, Inc.
  (PCSA of NM)**
Bear Canyon Senior Center
4645 Pitt NE
Albuquerque, NM 87108
505-254-7784
Meets on the first and third Saturdays of the month from 12:30
  to 2:30 PM

Belen Support Group
Affiliation: PCSA of NM
120 South 9th Street
Belen, NM
505-861-1013

Carlsbad Support
Affiliation: PCSA of NM
2522 West Pearse St.
Carlsbad, New Mexico
505-885-1557

Grants Support Group
Affiliation: PCSA of NM
Cibola Senior Center
1150 Elm Drive
Grants, NM
505-285-3922

Santa Fe Support Group
Affiliation: PCSA of NM
Meeting Location: Cancer Treatment Center of Santa Fe
455 St. Michaels Drive
Santa Fe, NM
505-466-4242

Socorro Support Group
Affiliation: PCSA of NM
Meeting Location: 1228 Hilton Place
Socorro, New Mexico
505-835-4766

Man to Man
Affiliation: American Cancer Society
95 Schwenk Drive
Kingston, NY
845-331-8300 or 800-233-5049
General meeting on the third Tuesday from 4:30 to 6:00 PM,
   Hurley Reformed Church Hall

Malecare
New York City, NY
212-844-8369
Meetings in several locations for spouse/partners, gays, transgen-
   dered
Monday: Men only, 6 PM, St. Vincent's Hospital Cancer,
   325 W. 15th
Tuesday: Men and Women, 5:30 PM, Lenox Hill Hospital,
   100 E. 77th, Conference Room 1
Tuesday: Men only, 7 PM, Beth Israel Hospital, 10 Union
   Square Eat 4th FL
Wednesday: Men and Women, 6 PM, New York Presbyterian
   Hospital, 16 W 60th, Suite 470

US TOO
Affiliation: Memorial Sloan Kettering/New York Presbyterian-
    Cornell Chapter
Memorial Sloan Kettering
Hoffman Auditorium
1275 New York Avenue
New York City, NY
212-717-3527
Meets on the third Thursday from 6 to 7 PM for the lecture and
    7:00 to 8:30 PM for the small group

Cancer Care, Inc.
275 7th Avenue
New York, NY
212-712-6121
Meets every first and third Tuesdays of the month from 5:30 to
    7:00 PM

Woodbury Long Island
Affiliation: Cancer Care of Long Island
20 Crossways Park North
Suite 110
Woodbury, NY
516-364-8130, ext. 106

US TOO Prostate Cancer Support Group of Wake County
Rex Cancer Center
Raleigh, NC
919-772-1047
Meets the second Thursday of the month at 7:00 PM

US TOO Prostate Support Group
Presbyterian Hospital
Raleigh, NC
704-563-9028

Wake County Prostate Cancer Support Group

Affiliations: American Cancer Society, US TOO, Rex Hospital
Rex Center
Cancer Center Auditorium, Raleigh
4420 Lake Boone, TX
919-846-8442
Meets from 7 to 9 PM on the second Thursday of the month
   except for December, July, and August

Cincinnati

Wellness Center
4918 Cooper Road
Cincinnati, OH
513-791-4060 or 513-321-1693
Small groups for men and women meet on the second Wednesday from 7 to 9 PM

James CCC PC Support Group

James Comprehensive Cancer Center
The Ohio State University
614-293-5066, 614-293-4646, or 800-293-5066
Meets the last Wednesday of each month: months alternate men
   only

US TOO of Central Oklahoma

Affiliation: US TOO
Oklahoma City, OK
405-604-4298
Meets on the third Monday from 6:00 to 7:30 PM; alternates
   between Deaconess Hospital and Integris Baptist Medical
Call for meeting locations

Florence Support Group

Affiliation: American Cancer Society
400 9th Street
Florence, OR
541-997-6626
Meets on the first Monday from 5:30 to 7:00 PM in Conference
   Room C, Peace Harbor Hospital

Amarillo PC Support Group
Meeting Location: Luby's Cafeteria on Coulter
Amarillo, TX
806-355-0806
Meets first Thursday of every third month from 6 to 8 PM

Dallas
A support group for gay men dealing with prostate cancer in the
    Dallas/Fort Worth/Mid-Cities area of North Texas
972-235-0257
Dallas, TX

Washington
Man to Man of Everett, WA
Affiliation: American Cancer Society
Meeting Location: Medical Building Colby Campus
14th and Colby
Everett, WA
360-568-2548
Meets on the third Wednesday from 7 to 9 PM; men only

Canada

Montréal West Island PC Support Group
Sarto Desnoyers Community Center
1335 Lake Shore Drive
Dorval, Québec
514-694-6412
Meets at 7:30 PM every fourth Thursday of the month except
    July, August, and December

Owen Sound (Ontario) PC Support Group
Affiliations: CPCN and US TOO
Meeting Location: St. Andrews Presbyterian Church
519-371-4779
Meets on the third Wednesday from 7 to 9 PM

Ireland

Men Against Cancer (MAC)
Sponsored by the Irish Cancer Society
c/o Irish Cancer Society
43/45 Northumberland Rd.
Dublin 4
FreeFone 1 800 200 700
Email: support
Website: www.cancer.ie/support/mac.php

Israel

You Are Not Alone (YANA)
Israeli Cancer Association, Building 5
Haifa, Israel
04-837-1733
Meets 6 PM on the last Thursday of every month, companions
  invited, meetings in Hebrew

South Africa

Wynberg Western Cape
Prostate Cancer Support Action (PSA) Group
Affiliation: National Cancer Association of South Africa
(021) 788-6280
Meets last Thursday of the month
Southern Cross Hospital, First Floor Seminar Room
Meets on the first Wednesday of the month from 11:30 AM to
  1:00 PM

Glossary

Acid phosphatase: Tumor marker for prostate cancer that is no longer used.

Alpha blockers: A class of drug used to treat prostate symptoms.

Alpha receptors: The nerve fibers that mediate bladder and prostate function and tone.

Alpha-1-antichymotrypsin: Substance in the blood that can bind PSA.

Anterior fibromuscular stoma: The front of the prostate gland.

Antiandrogen: Drugs that counteract the action of testosterone.

Azotemia: Increased serum creatinine which is a sign of kidney dysfunction.

Benign prostatic hypertrophy: A benign enlargement of the prostate

Bladder: The structure in the body that stores urine.

Bladder stones: Hard buildups of mineral that form in the urinary bladder.

Bladder ultrasound: A test done through the skin to measure how much urine is left in the bladder after voiding.

Brachycardia: A slow heart rate, usually under 60 beats per minute. A normal heart rate is from 60 to 100 beats per minute.

Bulbourethral glands: Two glands that discharge a component of seminal fluid into the urethra; also known as Cowper's glands.

Catheter: A soft plastic or rubber tube that is inserted in the urethra, through the prostate, and into the bladder in order to drain urine.

Central zone: The inner portion of the prostate.

Complexed PSA: PSA that is bound to alpha-1-antichymotrypsin.

Cryotherapy: Freezing the prostate as a cancer treatment.

Cystoscopy: A procedure to look into the bladder and urethra with a special tube.

Cystoscope: The instrument that is used to look into the bladder during a cystoscopy.

Diabetes mellitus: A disorder in which blood sugar (glucose) levels are abnormally high because the body does not produce enough insulin.

Digital rectal exam: Part of the physical exam where the urologist palpates the prostate by inserting a finger into the rectum.

Dihydrotestosterone: A metabolite of testosterone.

Electrovaporization: A procedure in which electric current is used to destroy prostate tissue.

Extravasation: A discharge or escape of fluid, normally found in a vessel or tube, into the surrounding tissue.

Free radical scavengers: Substances that can bind an atom or molecule with an unpaired electron.

Gene therapy: A technique used to correct defective genes.

Gonadotropin-releasing hormone: A hormone made by the hypothalamus that in turn stimulates the pituitary gland; abbreviated GnRH.

Hematospermia: The presence of blood in ejaculate (semen).

Hematuria: The presence of blood in urine.

Human glandular kallikrein: A substance made by the prostate gland that is not used as a tumor marker.

Hydronephrosis: Dilation of the kidneys, usually due to obstruction.

Hyponatremic: A low sodium level in the blood.

Impotence: The inability to achieve an erection or to maintain an erection until ejaculation.

Neurogenic bladder: A bladder that has an abnormality in its nerve supply.

Neurotransmitter: Chemicals that influence the function of nerves.

Nocturia: Getting up at night to urinate.

Norepinephrine: A neurotransmitter that regulates the sympathetic nervous system.

Open prostatectomy: A technique to remove the prostate through a skin incision.

Orchiectomy: Surgical removal of one or both testes.

Penis: The male organ used for urination and sexual intercourse.

Perineum: In a male, the region between the scrotum and rectum.

Peripheral zone: The posterior or back portion of the prostate.

Phytotherapy: The use of plants or plant extracts for medicinal purposes.

Postural hypotension: A drop in blood pressure upon standing.

Prostadynia: A spasm of the prostate that can cause symptoms similar to prostatitis.

Prostaglandins: Chemical messengers made by different organs in the body.

Prostate cancer: The most common male cancer, involving a malignant tumor growth in the prostate gland.

Prostate gland: A male gland that is located at the base of the bladder and surrounds the urethra.

Prostate-specific antigen (PSA): A chemical made by both benign and malignant prostate tissue. Measurement of PSA serum levels is used as a screening test for prostate cancer.

Prostatic stents: Cylindrical devices that can be placed in the urethra to relieve prostatic obstruction.

Prostatitis: An inflammation or infection of the prostate gland.

PSA density: A measurement calculated by dividing the serum PSA by the prostate volume.

PSA velocity: The change in the PSA level over time.

Radiation therapy: Radiation energy used to treat many types of cancer, usually administered over 6 to 7 weeks.

Radical prostatectomy: The surgical removal of the entire prostate and some of the surrounding tissue, done to treat prostate cancer.

Rectum: The final, straight portion of the large intestine, ending in the anus.

Resectionist: The physician (urologist) who use the resectoscope.

Resectoscope: An instrument used to remove (resect) prostate, bladder, or urethral tissue through the urethra.

Rhinitis: An inflammation of the nasal passages.

Seminal plasma: The majority of the ejaculatory fluid that is used to nourish the sperm.

Seminal vesicles: Two structures next to the prostate gland that contribute fluid to the ejaculate.

Serine protease: A class of peptidases found found in the blood.

Sperm: The cells in the male ejaculate that fertilize eggs.

Suprapubic prostatectomy: Removal of a portion of the prostate through a lower abdominal incision.

Suprapubic tube: A type of catheter placed percutaneously (through the skin) into the bladder through the lower abdominal wall in order to drain urine.

Testicles: The reproductive organs of the male, located in the scrotum.

Testosterone: The principal male sex hormone.

Transition zone: The area of the prostate that immediately surrounds the urethra.

Transrectal ultrasound: A procedure in which a probe is placed in the rectum to visualize the prostate.

Transurethral incision of the prostate: A method of removing prostatic obstruction using an incision instead of resection; also known as TUIP.

Transurethral prostatectomy: A method of removing obstructive prostate tissue through the urethra so that no external incision is made; also known as TURP.

Urethra: The tube that carries urine from the bladder to the outside of the body.

Urinary incontinence: Leakage of urine from the bladder through the urethra.

Urodynamics test: A test that assesses how well the bladder functions.

Uroflow: A measurement of the force and volume of the urine stream.

Urologist: A person trained to treat the genitourinary system.

Verumontanum: The area in the urethra where the ejaculatory ducts enter.

Index